Welcome to the ***"Gastric Bypass Surgery Cookbook: 110+ Nutritious Recipes for Post-Surgery Success."*** *If you're holding this book, you've likely undergone gastric bypass surgery or are preparing for it, embarking on a transformative journey toward improved health and well-being. This cookbook is designed to support you during this critical phase of your recovery by providing over 110 delicious and nourishing recipes tailored to meet your nutritional needs.*

Gastric bypass surgery is a significant step toward managing weight, improving overall health, and enhancing quality of life. Following surgery, it's essential to adopt dietary habits that support healing, promote weight loss, and prevent nutrient deficiencies. This cookbook is your guide to navigating the post-surgery dietary landscape, ensuring that you have access to flavorful meals that are not only nutritious but also satisfying.

The recipes in this cookbook are crafted with care to prioritize protein, vitamins, and minerals essential for your recovery and long-term health. Each recipe has been designed to be easy to prepare, using ingredients that are readily available and focusing on flavors that bring joy to your meals. Whether you're looking for hearty breakfasts, comforting soups, nourishing mains, or delightful desserts, you'll find a variety of options to suit your palate and dietary requirements.

In addition to delicious recipes, this book offers practical advice on meal planning, portion control, and navigating dietary changes after surgery. We understand that adjusting to a new way of eating can be challenging, and our goal is to provide you with the tools and support you need to succeed.

By embracing the recipes and principles outlined in this cookbook, you are taking proactive steps toward optimizing your health and achieving your wellness goals. We encourage you to approach this journey with patience, compassion for yourself, and a commitment to self-care through nutritious eating.

*Thank you for choosing the **"Gastric Bypass Surgery Cookbook"** as your companion on this transformative journey. We hope these recipes inspire you, nourish you, and contribute to your ongoing success and happiness as you embrace a healthier lifestyle post-surgery.*

Here's to your health, healing, and enjoying every flavorful bite along the way.

Let's get cooking!

Thank you for choosing the **"Gastric Bypass Surgery Cookbook: 110+ Nutritious Recipes for Post-Surgery Success."** Your decision to bring this book into your life signifies a commitment to your health and well-being, and we are truly grateful to be a part of your journey.

Navigating life after gastric bypass surgery can present its challenges, and we understand the importance of having access to delicious, nutritious meal options that support your recovery and long-term health goals. Each recipe in this cookbook has been carefully crafted to provide you with the essential nutrients your body needs, while also celebrating the joy of flavorful eating.

Your support means the world to us, and we hope that the recipes and guidance offered in this cookbook empower you on your path to success. Whether you're exploring new flavors, mastering cooking techniques, or simply enjoying meals that nourish both body and soul, we're here to support you every step of the way.

Once again, thank you for choosing the **"Gastric Bypass Surgery Cookbook."** We wish you continued health, happiness, and a future filled with delicious, nutritious meals that support your ongoing recovery and well-being.

Bon appétit and enjoy your culinary journey to post-surgery success!

Warm regards,

Daisy Robinson

1. Grilled chicken breast

Ingredient:

- 4 boneless, skinless chicken breasts (about 4•6 oz each)
- 1 tbsp olive oil
- 1 tsp garlic powder
- 1 tsp onion powder
- 1 tsp dried oregano
- Salt and pepper to taste

Instructions:

1. Preheat grill or grill pan to medium•high heat.

2. Brush the chicken breasts lightly with olive oil on both sides.

3. Season the chicken with garlic powder, onion powder, oregano, salt, and pepper.

4. Grill the chicken for 4•6 minutes per side, or until the internal temperature reaches 165°F.

5. Allow the chicken to rest for 5 minutes before serving.

Tips:
- Chicken breast is a lean protein that is easy to digest after gastric bypass surgery.

- Avoid heavy sauces or marinades that could be difficult to tolerate.

- Pair the grilled chicken with steamed vegetables or a small salad for a complete, gastric bypass•friendly meal.

- Be sure to chew the chicken thoroughly and eat slowly to prevent discomfort.

2. Baked fish (cod, salmon, tilapia)

Ingredient:

- 4 (4•6 oz) fish fillets (such as cod, salmon, or tilapia)
- 1 tbsp olive oil
- 1 tsp lemon juice
- 1 tsp dried dill
- 1/2 tsp garlic powder
- Salt and pepper to taste

Instructions:

1. Preheat oven to 400°F.

2. Place the fish fillets in a baking dish or on a parchment•lined baking sheet.

3. Drizzle the fish with olive oil and lemon juice, making sure to coat both sides.

4. Sprinkle the fish evenly with the dried dill, garlic powder, salt, and pepper.

5. Bake for 12•15 minutes, or until the fish flakes easily with a fork and reaches an internal temperature of 145°F.

6. Allow the fish to rest for 5 minutes before serving.

Tips:
- Fish is an excellent source of lean protein that is easy to digest after gastric bypass.

- Baking the fish keeps it moist and tender without the need for heavy sauces or breading.

- The lemon juice and dill add flavor without adding many calories or fat.

- Serve the baked fish with steamed vegetables or a small salad for a complete, gastric bypass•friendly meal.

- Be sure to chew the fish thoroughly and eat slowly to prevent discomfort.

3. Lean ground turkey patties

Ingredient:

- 1 lb lean ground turkey (93% lean or higher)
- 1 tsp garlic powder
- 1 tsp onion powder
- 1 tsp dried oregano
- 1/2 tsp salt
- 1/4 tsp black pepper

Instructions:

1. In a large bowl, gently mix together the ground turkey, garlic powder, onion powder, oregano, salt, and pepper until well combined.

2. Divide the mixture into 4 equal portions and shape each into a patty, about 4·5 inches wide and 1/2 inch thick.

3. Preheat a grill, grill pan, or non·stick skillet over medium·high heat.

4. Cook the turkey patties for 4·5 minutes per side, or until they are cooked through and reach an internal temperature of 165°F.

5. Allow the patties to rest for 5 minutes before serving.

Tips:
• Ground turkey is a lean protein that is easy to digest after gastric bypass surgery.

• Avoid adding any additional oils or fats to the patties, as they can be difficult to tolerate.

• The simple seasoning adds flavor without adding many calories or fat.

• Serve the turkey patties on their own or with a small side salad for a complete, gastric bypass·friendly meal.

• Be sure to chew the patties thoroughly and eat slowly to prevent discomfort.

4. Shrimp skewers

Ingredient:

- 1 lb large shrimp, peeled and deveined
- 1 tbsp olive oil
- 1 tsp lemon juice
- 1 tsp dried parsley
- 1/2 tsp garlic powder
- 1/4 tsp salt
- 1/4 tsp black pepper

Instructions:

1. Preheat grill or grill pan to medium•high heat.

2. In a medium bowl, toss the shrimp with the olive oil, lemon juice, dried parsley, garlic powder, salt, and pepper until evenly coated.

3. Thread the seasoned shrimp onto metal or wooden skewers, leaving a small space between each shrimp.

4. Grill the shrimp skewers for 2•3 minutes per side, or until the shrimp are opaque and cooked through.

5. Serve the grilled shrimp skewers immediately.

Tips:
- Shrimp is a lean protein that is easy to digest after gastric bypass surgery.

- The simple seasoning adds flavor without adding many calories or fat.

- Grilling the shrimp skewers keeps them moist and tender.

- Serve the shrimp skewers with a small salad or steamed vegetables for a complete, gastric bypass•friendly meal.

- Be sure to chew the shrimp thoroughly and eat slowly to prevent discomfort.

5. Hard•boiled eggs

Ingredient:

• 6 large eggs

Instructions:

1. Place the eggs in a single layer in a saucepan and cover with cold water by 1 inch.

2. Bring the water to a boil over high heat.

3. Once the water reaches a rolling boil, remove the pan from the heat and cover with a lid.

4. Let the eggs sit in the hot water for 12 minutes for hard•boiled eggs.

5. Drain the hot water and cover the eggs with cold water to stop the cooking process.

6. Let the eggs sit in the cold water for 5 minutes.

7. Peel the eggs and serve.

Tips:
• Hard•boiled eggs are a great source of lean protein that is easy to digest after gastric bypass surgery.

• Avoid adding any additional seasonings or sauces, as they can be difficult to tolerate.

• Serve the hard•boiled eggs on their own or with a small side salad for a complete, gastric bypass•friendly meal.

• Be sure to chew the eggs thoroughly and eat slowly to prevent discomfort.

6. Egg white omelet with vegetables

Ingredient:

- 4 large egg whites
- 1/4 cup diced bell pepper
- 1/4 cup diced onion
- 1/4 cup diced mushrooms
- 1 tbsp chopped fresh spinach
- 1 tsp olive oil
- Salt and pepper to taste

Instructions:

1. In a small bowl, whisk the egg whites until they are light and frothy.

2. Heat the olive oil in a non•stick skillet over medium heat.

3. Add the diced bell pepper, onion, and mushrooms to the skillet. Sauté for 2•3 minutes, or until the vegetables are tender.

4. Pour the whisked egg whites into the skillet and let them cook for 1•2 minutes, or until the bottom starts to set.

5. Sprinkle the chopped spinach over the egg whites and season with salt and pepper.

6. Using a spatula, gently fold the omelet in half and slide it onto a plate.

Tips:
- Egg whites are a lean protein that is easy to digest after gastric bypass surgery.

- The vegetables add fiber and nutrients without adding many calories or fat.

- Avoid adding any cheese or other high•fat toppings, as they can be difficult to tolerate.

- Serve the egg white omelet on its own or with a small side salad for a complete, gastric bypass•friendly meal.

- Be sure to chew the omelet thoroughly and eat slowly to prevent discomfort.

7. Tofu scramble

Ingredient:

- 1 block (14 oz) firm or extra•firm tofu, drained and crumbled
- 1 tbsp olive oil
- 1/2 cup diced onion
- 1/2 cup diced bell pepper
- 2 cloves garlic, minced
- 1 tsp ground cumin
- 1 tsp turmeric
- 1/4 tsp salt
- 1/4 tsp black pepper
- 2 tbsp chopped fresh parsley (optional)

Instructions:

1. Heat the olive oil in a non•stick skillet over medium heat.

2. Add the diced onion and bell pepper to the skillet. Sauté for 2•3 minutes, or until the vegetables are tender.

3. Add the minced garlic and sauté for an additional 1 minute.

4. Crumble the tofu into the skillet and stir to combine with the vegetables.

5. Sprinkle the ground cumin, turmeric, salt, and black pepper over the tofu mixture and stir to coat evenly.

6. Cook the tofu scramble for 5•7 minutes, stirring occasionally, until heated through.

7. Remove from heat and stir in the chopped parsley, if using.

8. Serve the tofu scramble warm.

Tips:
- Tofu is a lean, plant•based protein that is easy to digest after gastric bypass surgery.
- The vegetables add fiber and nutrients without adding many calories or fat.
- The spices add flavor without the need for high•fat sauces or toppings.
- Serve the tofu scramble on its own or with a small side of roasted vegetables for a complete, gastric bypass•friendly meal.
- Be sure to chew the tofu scramble thoroughly and eat slowly to prevent discomfort.

8. Cottage cheese with sliced cucumber

Ingredient:

- 1 cup low•fat or non•fat cottage cheese
- 1/2 cup sliced cucumber
- 1 tsp chopped fresh dill (optional)
- Salt and pepper to taste

Instructions:

1. In a small bowl, combine the cottage cheese and sliced cucumber.

2. If desired, sprinkle the chopped fresh dill over the top.

3. Season with a pinch of salt and pepper.

4. Serve immediately.

Tips:
- Cottage cheese is a great source of lean protein that is easy to digest after gastric bypass surgery.

- Cucumbers are a •calorie, high•fiber vegetable that can help promote feelings of fullness.

- The fresh dill adds a nice flavor without adding many calories or fat.

- This simple snack or side dish can be enjoyed on its own or with a small portion of grilled chicken or fish.

- Be sure to chew the cottage cheese and cucumber mixture thoroughly and eat slowly to prevent discomfort.

9. Greek yogurt with chia seeds

Ingredient:

• 1 cup plain, non•fat Greek yogurt
• 1 tbsp chia seeds
• 1/2 tsp vanilla extract (optional)
• Stevia or other no•calorie sweetener (optional)

Instructions:

1. In a small bowl, combine the Greek yogurt, chia seeds, and vanilla extract (if using).

2. Stir the mixture well to incorporate the chia seeds.

3. If desired, sweeten the yogurt with a small amount of stevia or other no•calorie sweetener.

4. Serve the Greek yogurt with chia seeds immediately.

Tips:
• Greek yogurt is a great source of protein that is easy to digest after gastric bypass surgery.

• Chia seeds are high in fiber, which can help promote feelings of fullness.

• The vanilla extract and sweetener (if using) add a touch of flavor without adding many calories or fat.

• This simple snack or breakfast can be enjoyed on its own or with a small portion of fresh berries.

• Be sure to chew the yogurt and chia seed mixture thoroughly and eat slowly to prevent discomfort.

10. Tuna salad (made with low•fat mayo)

Ingredient:

- 2 (5 oz) cans of water•packed tuna, drained
- 2 tbsp low•fat mayonnaise
- 1 tbsp plain, non•fat Greek yogurt
- 1 tsp Dijon mustard
- 1 tbsp finely chopped celery
- 1 tbsp finely chopped onion
- 1 tbsp chopped fresh parsley
- Salt and pepper to taste

Instructions:

1. In a medium bowl, combine the drained tuna, low•fat mayonnaise, Greek yogurt, and Dijon mustard. Stir until well mixed.

2. Fold in the chopped celery, onion, and parsley.

3. Season the tuna salad with salt and pepper to taste.

4. Serve the tuna salad on its own, on a bed of lettuce, or with a small portion of whole grain crackers or sliced cucumber.

Tips:
• Tuna is a lean protein that is easy to digest after gastric bypass surgery.

• Using a combination of low•fat mayonnaise and Greek yogurt helps reduce the overall fat and calorie content.

• The celery, onion, and parsley add flavor and crunch without adding many calories.

• Be sure to chew the tuna salad thoroughly and eat slowly to prevent discomfort.

• This tuna salad can be made in advance and stored in the refrigerator for up to 3 days.

11. Chicken salad (made with low•fat mayo)

Ingredient:

• 2 cups cooked, shredded chicken breast
• 2 tbsp low•fat mayonnaise
• 1 tbsp plain, non•fat Greek yogurt
• 1 tsp Dijon mustard
• 1 tbsp finely chopped celery
• 1 tbsp finely chopped onion
• 1 tbsp chopped fresh parsley
• Salt and pepper to taste

Instructions:

1. In a medium bowl, combine the shredded chicken, low•fat mayonnaise, Greek yogurt, and Dijon mustard. Stir until well mixed.

2. Fold in the chopped celery, onion, and parsley.

3. Season the chicken salad with salt and pepper to taste.

4. Serve the chicken salad on its own, on a bed of lettuce, or with a small portion of whole grain crackers or sliced cucumber.

Tips:
• Chicken is a lean protein that is easy to digest after gastric bypass surgery.

• Using a combination of low•fat mayonnaise and Greek yogurt helps reduce the overall fat and calorie content.

• The celery, onion, and parsley add flavor and crunch without adding many calories.

• Be sure to chew the chicken salad thoroughly and eat slowly to prevent discomfort.

• This chicken salad can be made in advance and stored in the refrigerator for up to 3 days.

12. Turkey roll•ups with lettuce and low•fat cheese

Ingredient:

• 8 slices of lean, deli•style turkey breast
• 4 leaves of romaine or green leaf lettuce
• 2 oz low•fat cheddar or Swiss cheese, sliced

Instructions:

1. Lay the turkey slices out flat on a clean surface.

2. Place a lettuce leaf on top of each turkey slice, trimming the lettuce to fit if needed.

3. Top each lettuce•wrapped turkey slice with a slice of low•fat cheese.

4. Carefully roll up the turkey, lettuce, and cheese into a tight roll.

5. Secure the roll•ups with toothpicks, if needed.

6. Slice each roll•up into 2•3 pieces and serve.

Tips:
• Turkey is a lean protein that is easy to digest after gastric bypass surgery.

• The lettuce and low•fat cheese provide additional nutrients without adding too many calories or fat.

• This recipe is simple and easy to prepare, making it a great option for a quick, gastric bypass•friendly snack or meal.

• Avoid any high•fat sauces or dressings, as they can be difficult to tolerate.

• Be sure to chew the roll•ups thoroughly and eat slowly to prevent discomfort.

13. Lean roast beef slices

Ingredient:

• 1 lb lean roast beef (look for cuts with "round" or "loin" in the name)
• 1 tsp garlic powder
• 1 tsp onion powder
• 1/2 tsp dried thyme
• 1/4 tsp salt
• 1/4 tsp black pepper

Instructions:

1. Preheat your oven to 375°F.

2. In a small bowl, combine the garlic powder, onion powder, dried thyme, salt, and black pepper.

3. Rub the seasoning mixture all over the roast beef.

4. Place the seasoned roast beef on a baking sheet or in a roasting pan.

5. Roast the beef for 25•30 minutes, or until it reaches an internal temperature of 145°F for medium•rare.

6. Allow the roast beef to rest for 5•10 minutes before slicing.

7. Slice the roast beef into thin, lean slices.

Tips:
• Lean roast beef is a great source of protein that is easy to digest after gastric bypass surgery.
• The simple seasoning adds flavor without adding many calories or fat.

• Avoid any high•fat sauces or gravies, as they can be difficult to tolerate.

• Serve the lean roast beef slices on their own or with a small side salad for a complete, gastric bypass•friendly meal.

• Be sure to chew the roast beef thoroughly and eat slowly to prevent discomfort.

14. Grilled pork tenderloin

Ingredient:

- 1 lb pork tenderloin
- 1 tbsp olive oil
- 1 tsp garlic powder
- 1 tsp onion powder
- 1 tsp dried thyme
- 1/2 tsp salt
- 1/4 tsp black pepper

Instructions:

1. Preheat your grill or grill pan to medium·high heat.

2. In a small bowl, combine the olive oil, garlic powder, onion powder, dried thyme, salt, and black pepper.

3. Rub the seasoning mixture all over the pork tenderloin.

4. Place the seasoned pork tenderloin on the preheated grill or grill pan.

5. Grill the pork for 12·15 minutes, turning occasionally, until it reaches an internal temperature of 145°F.

6. Remove the pork tenderloin from the grill and let it rest for 5·10 minutes before slicing.

7. Slice the pork tenderloin into thin, lean slices.

Tips:
- Pork tenderloin is a lean, tender cut of meat that is easy to digest after gastric bypass surgery.

- The simple seasoning adds flavor without adding many calories or fat.

- Avoid any high·fat sauces or marinades, as they can be difficult to tolerate.

- Serve the grilled pork tenderloin slices on their own or with a small side of roasted vegetables for a complete, gastric bypass·friendly meal.

- Be sure to chew the pork thoroughly and eat slowly to prevent discomfort.

15. Baked tofu cubes

Ingredient:

- 1 block (14 oz) firm or extra•firm tofu, drained and cut into 1•inch cubes
- 1 tbsp low•sodium soy sauce or tamari
- 1 tsp sesame oil
- 1 tsp rice vinegar
- 1 tsp garlic powder
- 1/2 tsp ground ginger
- 1/4 tsp black pepper

Instructions:

1. Preheat your oven to 400°F. Line a baking sheet with parchment paper.

2. In a medium bowl, whisk together the soy sauce, sesame oil, rice vinegar, garlic powder, ground ginger, and black pepper.

3. Add the tofu cubes to the bowl and gently toss to coat them evenly with the marinade.

4. Arrange the marinated tofu cubes in a single layer on the prepared baking sheet.

5. Bake the tofu for 20•25 minutes, flipping the cubes halfway through, until they are lightly browned and crispy on the outside.

6. Remove the baked tofu cubes from the oven and serve warm.

Tips:
- Tofu is a lean, plant•based protein that is easy to digest after gastric bypass surgery.

- The simple marinade adds flavor without the need for high•fat sauces or seasonings.

- Baking the tofu cubes gives them a crispy texture without frying.

- Serve the baked tofu cubes on their own or incorporate them into other gastric bypass•friendly dishes, such as salads or stir•fries.

- Be sure to chew the tofu thoroughly and eat slowly to prevent discomfort.

16. Low•fat string cheese

Ingredient:

• 1 serving (1 oz) low•fat string cheese

Instructions:

1. Unwrap the low•fat string cheese stick.

2. Slowly peel and pull the cheese into thin, stringy pieces, taking your time to chew each bite thoroughly.

That's it! This simple snack requires no preparation other than unwrapping the string cheese.

Tips for Enjoying Low•Fat String Cheese on a Gastric Bypass Diet:

• Choose low•fat or non•fat varieties of string cheese to keep the calorie and fat content low.
• Eat the string cheese slowly, taking small bites and chewing thoroughly to aid digestion.

• Pair the string cheese with a small serving of fresh vegetables, such as carrot sticks or cucumber slices, for added fiber and nutrients.

• Avoid any high•fat or sugary dips or toppings that could be difficult to tolerate.

• Stick to the recommended serving size of 1 oz (about 1 string cheese stick) to prevent overeating.

• Keep string cheese on hand for a quick, portable, and gastric bypass•friendly snack option.

17. Hummus with sliced bell peppers

Ingredient:

• 1/2 cup prepared, store•bought hummus (look for low•fat or reduced•calorie varieties)
• 1 medium bell pepper, sliced into strips

Instructions:

1. Scoop the hummus into a small serving bowl.

2. Arrange the sliced bell pepper strips around the hummus, using them as "dippers".

That's it! This simple snack requires no cooking, just assembly.

Tips for Enjoying Hummus and Bell Peppers on a Gastric Bypass Diet:

• Choose a hummus that is low in fat and calories, as high•fat dips can be difficult to tolerate after gastric bypass surgery.

• Bell peppers are a great source of fiber, vitamins, and minerals, and their crunchy texture pairs well with the smooth hummus.

• Avoid pairing the hummus with high•calorie or high•fat dippers like pita chips or crackers. Stick to the bell pepper strips.

• Eat the hummus and bell peppers slowly, taking small bites and chewing thoroughly to aid digestion.

• Portion control is key • stick to a 1/2 cup serving of hummus, which provides a good balance of protein and fiber.

• Prepare this snack in advance and store the hummus and bell pepper strips separately in the refrigerator for a quick, on•the•go option.

18. Edamame

Ingredient:

• 1 cup frozen, shelled edamame

Instructions:

1. Bring a small pot of water to a boil.

2. Add the frozen edamame to the boiling water and cook for 3•5 minutes, until heated through and tender.

3. Drain the edamame and transfer to a serving bowl.

4. Serve the edamame warm, with a sprinkle of salt if desired.

Tips for Enjoying Edamame on a Gastric Bypass Diet:

• Edamame is a great source of plant•based protein that is easy to digest after gastric bypass surgery.

• The pods can be a bit tough, so it's best to stick to the shelled variety, which is softer and easier to chew.

• Avoid adding any high•fat or high•sodium seasonings or sauces, as they can be difficult to tolerate.

• Eat the edamame slowly, taking small bites and chewing thoroughly to aid digestion.

• Pair the edamame with a small portion of another lean protein or non•starchy vegetable for a more complete, gastric bypass•friendly snack or meal.

• Edamame can be prepared in advance and stored in the refrigerator for a quick, on•the•go option.

19. Lentil soup

Ingredient:

- 1 cup dry brown or green lentils, rinsed
- 4 cups low•sodium vegetable or chicken broth
- 1 medium onion, diced
- 2 carrots, peeled and diced
- 2 celery stalks, diced
- 2 cloves garlic, minced
- 1 tsp dried thyme
- 1 bay leaf
- Salt and pepper to taste
- Chopped fresh parsley for garnish (optional)

Instructions:

1. In a large pot, combine the rinsed lentils and broth. Bring the mixture to a boil over high heat.

2. Reduce the heat to medium•low, then add the diced onion, carrots, celery, and minced garlic.

3. Stir in the dried thyme and bay leaf. Season with salt and pepper to taste.

4. Simmer the soup for 20•25 minutes, or until the lentils are tender and the vegetables are soft.

5. Remove the bay leaf. Ladle the lentil soup into bowls and garnish with chopped fresh parsley, if desired.

Tips:
- Lentils are a great source of lean protein and fiber, which can help promote feelings of fullness after gastric bypass surgery.
- Using low•sodium broth helps keep the sodium content in check.
- The simple vegetable and herb seasoning adds flavor without the need for high•fat ingredients.
- Serve the lentil soup on its own or with a small side salad for a complete, gastric bypass•friendly meal.
- Be sure to chew the soup thoroughly and eat slowly to prevent discomfort.

20. Black bean soup

Ingredient:

- 1 (15 oz) can low•sodium black beans, rinsed and drained
- 1 cup low•sodium vegetable or chicken broth
- 1/2 cup diced onion
- 1 clove garlic, minced
- 1 tsp ground cumin
- 1/4 tsp chili powder
- Salt and pepper to taste
- Chopped fresh cilantro for garnish (optional)

Instructions:

1. In a medium saucepan, combine the rinsed and drained black beans, broth, diced onion, and minced garlic.

2. Bring the mixture to a simmer over medium heat.

3. Stir in the ground cumin and chili powder. Season with salt and pepper to taste.

4. Reduce the heat to low and let the soup simmer for 10•15 minutes, stirring occasionally, until the flavors have melded and the soup has thickened slightly.

5. Ladle the black bean soup into bowls and garnish with chopped fresh cilantro, if desired.

Tips:
• Black beans are a great source of lean protein and fiber, which can help promote feelings of fullness after gastric bypass surgery.

• Using low•sodium broth and canned beans helps keep the sodium content in check.

• The simple seasoning adds flavor without the need for high•fat ingredients.

• Serve the black bean soup on its own or with a small side salad for a complete, gastric bypass•friendly meal.

• Be sure to chew the soup thoroughly and eat slowly to prevent discomfort.

21. Turkey chili

Ingredient:

• 1 lb ground turkey
• 1 medium onion, diced
• 2 cloves garlic, minced
• 1 (15 oz) can low•sodium diced tomatoes
• 1 (15 oz) can low•sodium black beans, rinsed and drained
• 1 (15 oz) can low•sodium kidney beans, rinsed and drained
• 2 tbsp chili powder
• 1 tsp ground cumin
• 1/2 tsp dried oregano
• 1/4 tsp cayenne pepper (optional)
• Salt and pepper to taste
• Chopped fresh cilantro for garnish (optional)

Instructions:

1. In a large pot or Dutch oven, cook the ground turkey over medium heat, breaking it up with a wooden spoon, until it is no longer pink, about 5•7 minutes.

2. Add the diced onion and minced garlic to the pot. Sauté for 2•3 minutes, until the onion is translucent.

3. Stir in the diced tomatoes, black beans, kidney beans, chili powder, cumin, oregano, and cayenne pepper (if using). Season with salt and pepper to taste.

4. Bring the chili to a simmer, then reduce the heat to low. Let the chili simmer for 15•20 minutes, stirring occasionally, to allow the flavors to meld.

5. Ladle the turkey chili into bowls and garnish with chopped fresh cilantro, if desired.

Tips:
• Ground turkey is a lean protein that is easy to digest after gastric bypass surgery.
• Using low•sodium canned beans and tomatoes helps keep the sodium content in check.
• The simple spices add flavor without the need for high•fat ingredients.
• Serve the turkey chili on its own or with a small side salad for a complete, gastric bypass•friendly meal.
• Be sure to chew the chili thoroughly and eat slowly to prevent discomfort.

22. Grilled shrimp with lemon and herbs

Ingredient:

- 1 lb large shrimp, peeled and deveined
- 2 tbsp olive oil
- 2 tbsp fresh lemon juice
- 1 tsp dried oregano
- 1 tsp dried basil
- 1/2 tsp garlic powder
- 1/4 tsp salt
- 1/4 tsp black pepper

Instructions:

1. Preheat your grill or grill pan to medium•high heat.

2. In a medium bowl, combine the shrimp, olive oil, lemon juice, oregano, basil, garlic powder, salt, and pepper. Toss to coat the shrimp evenly.

3. Thread the seasoned shrimp onto metal or wooden skewers, leaving a small space between each shrimp.

4. Grill the shrimp skewers for 2•3 minutes per side, or until the shrimp are opaque and cooked through.

5. Serve the grilled shrimp warm, with any remaining lemon juice and herb mixture drizzled over the top.

Tips:
- Shrimp is a lean protein that is easy to digest after gastric bypass surgery.
- The lemon, herbs, and simple seasoning add flavor without the need for high•fat sauces or marinades.
- Grilling the shrimp keeps them moist and tender, without the need for additional oils or fats.
- Serve the grilled shrimp on their own or with a side of steamed vegetables for a complete, gastric bypass•friendly meal.
- Be sure to chew the shrimp thoroughly and eat slowly to prevent discomfort.

23. Baked chicken tenders (using almond flour or whole wheat breadcrumbs)

Ingredient:

- 1 lb boneless, skinless chicken tenders
- 1 cup almond flour
- 1 tsp garlic powder
- 1 tsp onion powder
- 1/2 tsp paprika
- 1/4 tsp salt
- 1/4 tsp black pepper
- 1 tbsp olive oil

Instructions:

1. Preheat your oven to 400°F. Line a baking sheet with parchment paper.

2. In a shallow bowl, mix together the almond flour, garlic powder, onion powder, paprika, salt, and pepper.

3. Dredge the chicken tenders in the almond flour mixture, coating them evenly on all sides.

4. Place the coated chicken tenders on the prepared baking sheet. Drizzle the olive oil over the top.

5. Bake the chicken tenders for 18•22 minutes, flipping halfway through, until they are golden brown and cooked through.

6. Serve the baked almond flour chicken tenders warm.

Tips:
- Almond flour is a great gluten•free, low•carb coating option for individuals following a gastric bypass diet.
- The simple seasoning adds flavor without the need for high•fat sauces or breading.
- Baking the chicken tenders keeps them lean and easy to digest.
- Serve the chicken tenders on their own or with a side of roasted vegetables for a complete, gastric bypass•friendly meal.
- Be sure to chew the chicken thoroughly and eat slowly to prevent discomfort.

24. Sushi roll (tuna, salmon, or cucumber)

Ingredient:

- 1 cup cooked, short•grain brown rice
- 2 tbsp rice vinegar
- 1 tsp granulated sugar
- 1/4 tsp salt
- 1 cucumber, peeled, seeded, and cut into long, thin strips
- Nori seaweed sheets

Instructions:

1. In a small bowl, combine the cooked brown rice, rice vinegar, sugar, and salt. Stir until the sugar and salt have dissolved.

2. Lay a sheet of nori seaweed on a bamboo sushi mat or clean, flat surface. Spread about 1/2 cup of the seasoned rice evenly over the nori, leaving a 1•inch border at the top.

3. Arrange the cucumber strips in a line across the center of the rice.

4. Carefully roll the nori and rice around the cucumber, using the sushi mat to help you roll it tightly. Moisten the top edge of the nori with a bit of water to help it seal.

5. Slice the rolled sushi into 6•8 pieces using a sharp, wet knife.

6. Serve the cucumber sushi rolls immediately, with low•sodium soy sauce or wasabi on the side, if desired.

Tips:
- Cucumber is a low•calorie, high•fiber vegetable that is easy to digest after gastric bypass surgery.
- Brown rice provides complex carbohydrates and fiber, which can help promote feelings of fullness.
- Avoid using raw fish or high•fat fillings, as they may be difficult to tolerate.
- Be sure to chew the sushi rolls thoroughly and eat slowly to prevent discomfort.
- This recipe can also be adapted to use tuna or salmon as the filling, if desired.

25. Canned salmon with low•fat crackers

Ingredient:

• 1 (5 oz) can of wild•caught salmon, drained
• 1•2 tbsp low•fat mayonnaise or plain, non•fat Greek yogurt (optional)
• 8•10 whole grain, low•fat crackers

Instructions:

1. In a small bowl, flake the drained canned salmon with a fork.

2. If desired, mix in 1•2 tablespoons of low•fat mayonnaise or plain, non•fat Greek yogurt to bind the salmon together.

3. Serve the salmon salad with the low•fat crackers on the side.

Tips for Enjoying Canned Salmon and Crackers on a Gastric Bypass Diet:

• Canned salmon is a great source of lean protein that is easy to digest after gastric bypass surgery.

• Choose low•fat or reduced•calorie mayonnaise or Greek yogurt to keep the fat and calorie content in check.

• Opt for whole grain, low•fat crackers that are low in calories and carbohydrates.

• Avoid any high•fat or high•sodium crackers, as they can be difficult to tolerate.

• Eat the salmon and crackers slowly, taking small bites and chewing thoroughly to aid digestion.

• This snack can be prepared in advance and stored in the refrigerator for a quick, on•the•go option.

• Pair the salmon and crackers with a small serving of fresh vegetables for added fiber and nutrients.

26. Protein smoothie
(using protein powder, low•fat milk, and frozen berries)

Ingredient:

• 1 scoop (about 25•30 grams) unflavored or vanilla protein powder
• 1 cup unsweetened almond milk or low•fat dairy milk
• 1/2 cup frozen mixed berries
• 1 tbsp ground flaxseed (optional)
• 1 tsp honey or maple syrup (optional)
• Ice cubes (optional)

Instructions:

1. Add the protein powder, milk, frozen berries, and flaxseed (if using) to a high•powered blender.

2. Blend the ingredients on high speed until smooth and creamy, about 30 seconds to 1 minute.

3. If a thicker consistency is desired, add a few ice cubes and blend again briefly.

4. Taste the smoothie and add a teaspoon of honey or maple syrup if you'd like it to be slightly sweeter.

5. Pour the protein smoothie into a glass and enjoy immediately.

Tips:
• Protein powder provides a concentrated source of lean protein to help meet your needs after gastric bypass surgery.

• Unsweetened almond milk or low•fat dairy milk are good options that are easy to digest.
• Frozen berries add natural sweetness, fiber, and antioxidants without adding many calories.

• Ground flaxseed provides additional fiber and healthy fats.

• Avoid adding high•calorie or high•fat ingredients like peanut butter, ice cream, or full•fat dairy.

• Sip the smoothie slowly and chew any solid pieces thoroughly to prevent discomfort.

27. Egg salad (made with low•fat mayo)

Ingredient:

- 6 hard•boiled eggs, peeled and chopped
- 2 tbsp low•fat mayonnaise
- 1 tbsp plain, non•fat Greek yogurt
- 1 tsp Dijon mustard
- 1 tbsp finely chopped celery
- 1 tbsp finely chopped onion
- 1 tbsp chopped fresh parsley
- Salt and pepper to taste

Instructions:

1. In a medium bowl, combine the chopped hard•boiled eggs, low•fat mayonnaise, Greek yogurt, and Dijon mustard. Stir until well mixed.

2. Fold in the chopped celery, onion, and parsley.

3. Season the egg salad with salt and pepper to taste.

4. Serve the egg salad on its own, on a bed of lettuce, or with a small portion of whole grain crackers or sliced cucumber.

Tips:
- Hard•boiled eggs are a lean protein that is easy to digest after gastric bypass surgery.

- Using a combination of low•fat mayonnaise and Greek yogurt helps reduce the overall fat and calorie content.

- The celery, onion, and parsley add flavor and crunch without adding many calories.

- Be sure to chew the egg salad thoroughly and eat slowly to prevent discomfort.

- This egg salad can be made in advance and stored in the refrigerator for up to 3 days.

28. Grilled chicken skewers with vegetables

Ingredient:

• 1 lb boneless, skinless chicken breasts, cut into 1•inch cubes
• 1 red bell pepper, cut into 1•inch pieces
• 1 zucchini, cut into 1•inch pieces
• 1 red onion, cut into 1•inch pieces
• 2 tbsp olive oil
• 1 tsp garlic powder
• 1 tsp dried oregano
• 1/2 tsp salt
• 1/4 tsp black pepper

Instructions:

1. Preheat your grill or grill pan to medium•high heat.

2. In a large bowl, combine the cubed chicken, bell pepper, zucchini, and red onion. Drizzle with the olive oil and sprinkle with the garlic powder, dried oregano, salt, and black pepper. Toss to coat the ingredients evenly.

3. Thread the seasoned chicken and vegetables onto metal or wooden skewers, alternating the ingredients.

4. Grill the skewers for 12•15 minutes, turning occasionally, until the chicken is cooked through and the vegetables are tender.

5. Serve the grilled chicken and vegetable skewers immediately.

Tips:
• Chicken is a lean protein that is easy to digest after gastric bypass surgery.

• The vegetables add fiber, vitamins, and minerals without adding many calories or fat.

• The simple seasoning adds flavor without the need for high•fat sauces or marinades.

• Grilling the skewers keeps the ingredients moist and tender.

• Serve the grilled chicken and vegetable skewers on their own or with a small side salad for a complete, gastric bypass•friendly meal.Be sure to chew the skewers thoroughly and eat slowly to prevent discomfort.

29. Baked turkey meatballs

Ingredient:

- 1 lb ground turkey
- 1/4 cup whole wheat breadcrumbs or almond flour
- 1 egg, lightly beaten
- 2 tbsp grated Parmesan cheese
- 2 cloves garlic, minced
- 1 tsp dried oregano
- 1/2 tsp salt
- 1/4 tsp black pepper

Instructions:

1. Preheat your oven to 400°F. Line a baking sheet with parchment paper.

2. In a large bowl, combine the ground turkey, breadcrumbs or almond flour, egg, Parmesan cheese, minced garlic, dried oregano, salt, and black pepper. Mix until the ingredients are well incorporated.

3. Scoop the turkey mixture by the tablespoon and roll it into small, 1·inch meatballs. Place the meatballs on the prepared baking sheet, spacing them apart.

4. Bake the turkey meatballs for 18·22 minutes, or until they are cooked through and lightly browned.

5. Serve the baked turkey meatballs warm, on their own or with a small portion of marinara sauce or low·fat cheese.

Tips:
- Ground turkey is a lean protein that is easy to digest after gastric bypass surgery.
- Whole wheat breadcrumbs or almond flour provide a low·carb, gluten·free binder for the meatballs.
- The Parmesan cheese and simple seasoning add flavor without the need for high·fat ingredients.
- Baking the meatballs keeps them lean and easy to digest.
- Serve the turkey meatballs on their own or with a side of roasted vegetables for a complete, gastric bypass·friendly meal.
- Be sure to chew the meatballs thoroughly and eat slowly to prevent discomfort.

30. Chicken vegetable soup

Ingredient:

- 1 lb boneless, skinless chicken breasts, cut into 1·inch pieces
- 1 tablespoon olive oil
- 1 onion, diced
- 3 carrots, peeled and sliced
- 3 celery stalks, sliced
- 3 cloves garlic, minced
- 6 cups low·sodium chicken broth
- 2 bay leaves
- 1 teaspoon dried thyme
- 1 teaspoon dried oregano
- Salt and pepper to taste
- 2 cups chopped kale or spinach
- 1 cup frozen peas
- 1/4 cup chopped fresh parsley

Instructions:

1. In a large pot or Dutch oven, heat the olive oil over medium heat. Add the chicken and cook for 3·4 minutes until lightly browned.

2. Add the onion, carrots, celery and garlic. Cook for 5 minutes, stirring occasionally, until the vegetables start to soften.

3. Pour in the chicken broth and add the bay leaves, thyme, oregano, salt and pepper. Bring to a boil.

4. Reduce heat and let the soup simmer for 15·20 minutes, until the chicken is cooked through and the vegetables are tender.

5. Stir in the kale/spinach, peas and parsley. Cook for 5 more minutes.

6. Taste and adjust seasonings as needed.

7. Serve hot. Enjoy!

31. Steamed fish with ginger and scallions

Ingredient:

• 1 lb white fish fillets (such as tilapia, cod or halibut), cut into 4 portions
• 2 tablespoons low•sodium soy sauce
• 1 tablespoon rice vinegar
• 1 teaspoon sesame oil
• 2 teaspoons grated fresh ginger
• 3 scallions, thinly sliced
• Salt and pepper to taste

Instructions:

1. Set up a steamer basket in a pot with about 1 inch of water in the bottom. Bring the water to a boil.

2. In a small bowl, whisk together the soy sauce, rice vinegar, sesame oil and ginger.

3. Place the fish fillets in the steamer basket. Pour the soy sauce mixture over the top and sprinkle with the sliced scallions.

4. Steam the fish for 8•10 minutes, until it flakes easily with a fork.

5. Transfer the fish to a serving plate. Season with a pinch of salt and pepper.

6. Serve the fish hot, with the steaming liquid spooned over the top.

This dish is perfect for a gastric bypass diet as it is low in calories, high in protein, and easy to digest. The ginger and scallions add lots of flavor without the need for heavy sauces or seasonings. Enjoy!

32. Grilled tofu steaks with low•sodium soy sauce

Ingredient:

- 1 block (14 oz) extra•firm tofu, cut into 4 thick "steaks"
- 2 tablespoons low•sodium soy sauce
- 1 tablespoon rice vinegar
- 1 teaspoon sesame oil
- 1 teaspoon honey
- 1 clove garlic, minced
- 1/2 teaspoon ground ginger
- Salt and pepper to taste
- Cooking spray or oil for grilling

Instructions:

1. Pat the tofu steaks dry with paper towels. Place them on a plate or baking sheet.

2. In a small bowl, whisk together the low•sodium soy sauce, rice vinegar, sesame oil, honey, garlic and ground ginger.

3. Brush or spoon the soy sauce mixture evenly over both sides of the tofu steaks. Let marinate for 15•20 minutes.

4. Preheat grill or grill pan to medium•high heat. Lightly spray or oil the grates.

5. Carefully place the marinated tofu steaks on the hot grill. Cook for 4•5 minutes per side, until grill marks appear and the tofu is heated through.

6. Transfer the grilled tofu steaks to a plate. Season with a pinch of salt and pepper.

7. Serve the tofu steaks warm, with any remaining soy sauce mixture drizzled over the top.

This grilled tofu dish is a great protein•packed option for a gastric bypass diet. The low•sodium soy sauce and minimal oil keep it light and easy to digest. Enjoy!

33. Egg and vegetable frittata

Ingredient:

- 8 large eggs
- 1/4 cup unsweetened almond milk (or low•fat milk)
- 1/4 teaspoon salt
- 1/4 teaspoon black pepper
- 1 tablespoon olive oil
- 1 cup diced bell peppers
- 1 cup diced zucchini
- 1/2 cup diced onion
- 2 cloves garlic, minced
- 1/2 cup shredded low•fat cheddar cheese (optional)
- 2 tablespoons chopped fresh herbs (such as parsley, basil or chives)

Instructions:

1. Preheat oven to 375°F. Grease a 9•inch pie dish or oven•safe skillet with nonstick cooking spray.

2. In a large bowl, whisk together the eggs, almond milk, salt and pepper until well combined.

3. In a skillet over medium heat, heat the olive oil. Add the bell peppers, zucchini, onion and garlic. Sauté for 5•7 minutes, until the vegetables are tender.

4. Pour the egg mixture over the cooked vegetables in the skillet. Top with the shredded cheese, if using.

5. Transfer the skillet to the preheated oven. Bake for 18•22 minutes, until the center is set and the edges are lightly browned.

6. Remove the frittata from the oven and let cool for 5 minutes. Sprinkle with the chopped fresh herbs.

7. Slice and serve the frittata warm. Enjoy!

This frittata is packed with protein from the eggs and nutrients from the vegetables, making it a great option for a gastric bypass diet. The low•fat cheese is optional, but adds a nice creaminess. Adjust the vegetables to your liking.

34. Turkey burger with whole wheat bun

Ingredient:

- 1 lb ground turkey breast
- 1 egg white
- 1/4 cup whole wheat breadcrumbs
- 1 tablespoon Dijon mustard
- 1 teaspoon dried oregano
- 1/2 teaspoon garlic powder
- 1/4 teaspoon salt
- 1/4 teaspoon black pepper
- 4 whole wheat hamburger buns
- Toppings of your choice (such as lettuce, tomato, onion, pickles)

Instructions:

1. In a large bowl, combine the ground turkey, egg white, breadcrumbs, mustard, oregano, garlic powder, salt and pepper. Mix gently until just combined, being careful not to overmix.

2. Divide the turkey mixture into 4 equal portions and shape into patties, about 4·5 inches wide and 1/2 inch thick.

3. Preheat a grill or grill pan over medium·high heat. Lightly spray or oil the grates.

4. Cook the turkey burgers for 4·5 minutes per side, until cooked through and no longer pink in the center. An instant·read thermometer should read 165°F.

5. Toast the whole wheat buns on the grill or in a toaster.

6. Place the cooked turkey burgers on the toasted buns. Top with your desired toppings.

7. Serve the turkey burgers immediately, while hot.

This turkey burger is a great option for a gastric bypass diet. The lean turkey provides protein, while the whole wheat bun offers complex carbs and fiber. Feel free to load it up with your favorite fresh veggies for added nutrients.

35. Grilled chicken Caesar salad (with low•fat dressing)

Ingredient:

For the Salad:
• 4 boneless, skinless chicken breasts
• 1 romaine lettuce heart, chopped
• 1 cup cherry tomatoes, halved
• 1/2 cup shredded low•fat mozzarella cheese
• 2 tablespoons grated Parmesan cheese
• Croutons (optional)

For the Low•Fat Caesar Dressing:
• 1/4 cup plain Greek yogurt
• 2 tablespoons low•fat mayonnaise
• 2 tablespoons lemon juice
• 1 garlic clove, minced
• 1 teaspoon Dijon mustard
• 1/4 teaspoon Worcestershire sauce
• Salt and pepper to taste

Instructions:

1. Preheat grill or grill pan to medium•high heat. Season the chicken breasts with salt and pepper.

2. Grill the chicken for 5•7 minutes per side, until cooked through. Let rest for 5 minutes, then slice or chop the chicken.

3. In a small bowl, whisk together all the dressing ingredients until well combined.

4. In a large salad bowl, combine the chopped romaine, tomatoes, mozzarella, Parmesan and grilled chicken.

5. Drizzle the low•fat Caesar dressing over the salad and toss gently to coat.

6. Top the salad with croutons, if desired. Serve immediately.

This grilled chicken Caesar salad is a great option for a gastric bypass diet. The lean protein from the chicken, fiber from the greens, and creamy low•fat dressing make it a nutritious and satisfying meal. Adjust the amounts to suit your appetite.

36. Steamed broccoli

Ingredient:

- 1 lb broccoli florets
- 1•2 tablespoons water
- Salt and pepper to taste (optional)

Instructions:

1. Fill a medium saucepan with about 1 inch of water. Bring the water to a boil over high heat.

2. Place the broccoli florets in a steamer basket or colander that fits inside the saucepan. Make sure the water doesn't touch the bottom of the steamer.

3. Cover the saucepan with a lid and steam the broccoli for 5•7 minutes, until tender•crisp. The broccoli should be bright green and easily pierced with a fork.

4. Carefully remove the steamer basket or colander from the saucepan. Transfer the steamed broccoli to a serving bowl.

5. If desired, season the broccoli with a pinch of salt and pepper.

6. Serve the steamed broccoli warm.

Tips:
• For extra flavor, you can drizzle the broccoli with a bit of lemon juice or low•sodium soy sauce.
• Avoid overcooking the broccoli, as it can become mushy.
• Steaming is a great cooking method for gastric bypass patients as it preserves nutrients and is easy to digest.

This simple steamed broccoli dish is a great side option that is low in calories, high in fiber and nutrients, and gentle on the digestive system • perfect for a gastric bypass diet.

37. Roasted asparagus

Ingredient:

- 1 lb asparagus, tough ends trimmed
- 1 tablespoon olive oil
- 1/4 teaspoon salt
- 1/4 teaspoon black pepper

Instructions:

1. Preheat your oven to 400°F (200°C).

2. Wash the asparagus and pat it dry with paper towels. Trim off the tough, woody ends of the asparagus spears.

3. Arrange the asparagus spears in a single layer on a large baking sheet. Drizzle the olive oil over the asparagus and use your hands to gently toss and coat the spears.

4. Sprinkle the salt and black pepper evenly over the asparagus.

5. Roast the asparagus in the preheated oven for 12•15 minutes, flipping halfway through, until the asparagus is tender and lightly browned.

6. Remove the roasted asparagus from the oven and transfer it to a serving dish.

Tips:
- For even cooking, try to choose asparagus spears that are similar in thickness.
- Adjust the roasting time based on the thickness of your asparagus spears. Thinner spears may need less time.
- You can also add a squeeze of lemon juice or a sprinkle of grated Parmesan cheese for extra flavor.

Roasted asparagus is a fantastic side dish option for a gastric bypass diet. It's low in calories, high in fiber and nutrients, and the roasting process brings out the natural sweetness of the asparagus. Enjoy!

38. Grilled zucchini

Ingredient:

- 2 medium zucchini, sliced into 1/4•inch thick rounds
- 1 tablespoon olive oil
- 1/2 teaspoon garlic powder
- 1/4 teaspoon salt
- 1/4 teaspoon black pepper

Instructions:

1. Preheat your grill or grill pan to medium•high heat.

2. In a large bowl, toss the zucchini slices with the olive oil, garlic powder, salt, and black pepper until the zucchini is evenly coated.

3. Arrange the seasoned zucchini slices in a single layer on the preheated grill or grill pan.

4. Grill the zucchini for 3•4 minutes per side, or until tender and lightly charred.

5. Use tongs to transfer the grilled zucchini slices to a serving plate.

Tips:
• For best results, choose firm, fresh zucchini that is free of blemishes.

• You can also use a grill basket or aluminum foil with holes poked in it to prevent the zucchini from falling through the grates.

• Adjust the grilling time based on the thickness of your zucchini slices. Thinner slices may cook faster.

• Feel free to experiment with different seasonings, such as lemon zest, Italian herbs, or a sprinkle of Parmesan cheese.

Grilled zucchini is a simple, healthy, and delicious side dish that is perfect for a gastric bypass diet. The grilling process brings out the natural sweetness of the zucchini while keeping it tender and easy to digest.

39. Sautéed spinach

Ingredient:

• 1 lb fresh spinach, washed and stems removed
• 1 tablespoon olive oil
• 2 cloves garlic, minced
• 1/4 teaspoon salt
• 1/8 teaspoon black pepper

Instructions:

1. In a large skillet or sauté pan, heat the olive oil over medium heat.

2. Add the minced garlic to the hot oil and cook for 30 seconds to 1 minute, until fragrant.

3. Add the fresh spinach to the pan in batches, if needed, and sauté for 2•3 minutes, stirring frequently, until the spinach is wilted and tender.

4. Season the sautéed spinach with salt and black pepper. Taste and adjust seasoning as needed.

5. Serve the sautéed spinach warm.

Tips:
• For best texture, avoid overcooking the spinach. It should be tender but still bright green.

• You can add a squeeze of lemon juice or a sprinkle of grated Parmesan cheese for extra flavor.

• If the spinach seems dry, you can add a tablespoon or two of water or low•sodium broth to the pan.

• This recipe works well with other greens like kale, Swiss chard, or collard greens.

Sautéed spinach is a nutrient•dense, low•calorie side dish that's perfect for a gastric bypass diet. The quick cooking method helps preserve the spinach's vitamins and minerals, making it an easy and healthy option.

40. Mashed cauliflower

Ingredient:

- 1 large head of cauliflower, cut into florets (about 4 cups)
- 2 tablespoons unsweetened almond milk (or low•fat milk)
- 1 tablespoon butter or olive oil
- 1/4 teaspoon garlic powder
- 1/4 teaspoon salt
- 1/8 teaspoon black pepper

Instructions:

1. In a large pot, bring 1•2 inches of water to a boil. Add the cauliflower florets, cover, and steam for 8•10 minutes, until very tender.

2. Drain the cauliflower and transfer it to a food processor or high•powered blender.

3. Add the almond milk, butter/olive oil, garlic powder, salt, and black pepper to the food processor.

4. Blend or process the cauliflower mixture until smooth and creamy, scraping down the sides as needed.

5. Taste and adjust seasoning as desired, adding more salt, pepper, or garlic powder to your preference.

6. Transfer the mashed cauliflower to a serving bowl and serve warm.

Tips:
- For a creamier texture, you can add an extra tablespoon or two of almond milk.
- Experiment with different herbs and spices, such as rosemary, thyme, or chives.
- You can also stir in a tablespoon of grated Parmesan cheese for extra flavor.
- Mashed cauliflower can be made ahead of time and reheated gently before serving.

Mashed cauliflower is a fantastic low•carb, low•calorie alternative to traditional mashed potatoes. It's packed with fiber, vitamins, and minerals, making it a great option for a gastric bypass diet. Enjoy!

41. Baked sweet potato

Ingredient:

- 4 medium sweet potatoes, scrubbed clean
- 1 teaspoon olive oil
- 1/4 teaspoon salt
- 1/8 teaspoon black pepper

Instructions:

1. Preheat your oven to 400°F (200°C).

2. Use a fork to poke several holes all over the sweet potatoes. This will allow steam to escape during baking.

3. Rub the outside of the sweet potatoes lightly with the olive oil and sprinkle with the salt and pepper.

4. Place the sweet potatoes directly on the oven rack or on a baking sheet lined with parchment paper.

5. Bake the sweet potatoes for 45•60 minutes, until they are very tender when pierced with a fork. The cooking time may vary depending on the size of the sweet potatoes.

6. Remove the baked sweet potatoes from the oven and let them cool for 5 minutes.

7. Slice the sweet potatoes open lengthwise and fluff the insides with a fork.

8. Serve the baked sweet potatoes warm, with any desired toppings such as a sprinkle of cinnamon, a drizzle of honey, or a dollop of plain Greek yogurt.

Tips:
- For even cooking, try to choose sweet potatoes that are similar in size.
- You can also cut the sweet potatoes in half lengthwise before baking for faster cooking.
- Baked sweet potatoes can be made ahead of time and reheated gently before serving.

Baked sweet potatoes are an excellent source of fiber, vitamins, and complex carbohydrates, making them a great option for a gastric bypass diet. Enjoy this simple and nutritious side dish!

42. Quinoa pilaf

Ingredient:

- 1 cup uncooked quinoa, rinsed
- 2 cups low•sodium chicken or vegetable broth
- 1 tablespoon olive oil
- 1 small onion, diced
- 2 cloves garlic, minced
- 1 cup diced bell peppers (any color)
- 1/2 cup diced zucchini or yellow squash
- 1/4 cup chopped fresh parsley
- 1/4 teaspoon salt
- 1/4 teaspoon black pepper

Instructions:

1. In a medium saucepan, combine the rinsed quinoa and broth. Bring to a boil over high heat.

2. Once boiling, reduce the heat to low, cover the pan with a lid, and simmer for 15•20 minutes, until the quinoa is tender and the liquid is absorbed.

3. While the quinoa is cooking, heat the olive oil in a skillet over medium heat. Add the diced onion and sauté for 2•3 minutes until translucent.

4. Add the minced garlic, diced bell peppers, and diced zucchini/squash to the skillet. Sauté for an additional 5 minutes, until the vegetables are tender.

5. Fluff the cooked quinoa with a fork and transfer it to a large bowl. Add the sautéed vegetables, chopped parsley, salt, and pepper. Stir to combine. Serve the quinoa pilaf warm. Enjoy!

Tips:
- For extra flavor, you can add a squeeze of lemon juice or a sprinkle of grated Parmesan cheese.
- Feel free to customize the vegetables based on your preferences or what you have on hand.
- Quinoa is a great source of protein, fiber, and complex carbohydrates, making it an excellent choice for a gastric bypass diet.

This quinoa pilaf is a nutritious and versatile side dish that's easy to digest and packed with beneficial nutrients. Enjoy!

43. Brown rice

Ingredient:

• 1 cup uncooked brown rice
• 2 cups low•sodium chicken or vegetable broth
• 1/4 teaspoon salt (optional)

Instructions:

1. Rinse the brown rice in a fine•mesh strainer until the water runs clear. This helps remove any excess starch.

2. In a medium saucepan, combine the rinsed brown rice, broth, and salt (if using). Bring the mixture to a boil over high heat.

3. Once boiling, reduce the heat to low, cover the saucepan with a tight•fitting lid, and simmer for 45•50 minutes, until the rice is tender and the liquid is absorbed.

4. Remove the saucepan from the heat and let the brown rice sit, covered, for 5•10 minutes.

5. Fluff the cooked brown rice with a fork before serving.

Tips:
• For extra flavor, you can add a bay leaf, garlic, or herbs to the cooking liquid.
• Brown rice has a slightly nutty, chewy texture compared to white rice. It's higher in fiber, vitamins, and minerals.

• Cooked brown rice can be stored in the refrigerator for 3•5 days or frozen for up to 3 months.

• Adjust the cooking time as needed based on the type of brown rice you're using (short, medium, or long grain).

Brown rice is a great whole grain option for a gastric bypass diet. It's high in fiber, which can help promote feelings of fullness, and it's easy to digest. Enjoy it as a side dish or use it in other recipes.

44. Whole wheat couscous

Ingredient:

- 1 cup uncooked whole wheat couscous
- 1 1/4 cups low•sodium chicken or vegetable broth
- 1/4 teaspoon salt (optional)

Instructions:

1. In a medium saucepan, bring the broth and salt (if using) to a boil over high heat.

2. Once boiling, remove the saucepan from the heat and stir in the uncooked whole wheat couscous.

3. Cover the saucepan with a lid and let the couscous sit for 5•7 minutes, until all the liquid has been absorbed.

4. Fluff the cooked couscous with a fork, breaking up any clumps.

5. Serve the whole wheat couscous warm, or let it cool and then refrigerate for later use.

Tips:
- For extra flavor, you can add herbs, spices, or a squeeze of lemon juice to the couscous.
- Whole wheat couscous has a slightly nuttier and chewier texture compared to regular couscous.
- Cooked couscous can be stored in the refrigerator for 3•4 days or frozen for up to 3 months.
- Couscous is a quick•cooking whole grain that is easy to digest, making it a great option for a gastric bypass diet.

Whole wheat couscous is a versatile and nutritious whole grain that can be used as a side dish or incorporated into other recipes. It's high in fiber and complex carbohydrates, which can help keep you feeling full and satisfied.

45. Roasted Brussels sprouts

Ingredient:

• 1 lb Brussels sprouts, trimmed and halved
• 1 tablespoon olive oil
• 1/4 teaspoon salt
• 1/8 teaspoon black pepper

Instructions:

1. Preheat your oven to 400°F (200°C).

2. In a large bowl, toss the trimmed and halved Brussels sprouts with the olive oil, salt, and black pepper until the sprouts are evenly coated.

3. Spread the seasoned Brussels sprouts in a single layer on a large baking sheet or rimmed baking dish.

4. Roast the Brussels sprouts in the preheated oven for 20•25 minutes, tossing halfway through, until they are tender and lightly browned.

5. Remove the roasted Brussels sprouts from the oven and transfer them to a serving dish.

Tips:
• For even cooking, try to cut the Brussels sprouts into similar•sized pieces.

• You can also add other seasonings, such as garlic powder, paprika, or a sprinkle of Parmesan cheese.

• Roasting brings out the natural sweetness of the Brussels sprouts and makes them deliciously crispy on the outside.

• Roasted Brussels sprouts can be served as a side dish or incorporated into other recipes, such as salads or grain bowls.

Brussels sprouts are an excellent source of fiber, vitamins, and minerals, making them a great choice for a gastric bypass diet. The roasting process makes them easy to digest and full of flavor.

46. Steamed green beans

Ingredient:

• 1 lb fresh green beans, trimmed
• 1•2 tablespoons water
• Salt and pepper to taste (optional)

Instructions:

1. Fill a medium saucepan with about 1 inch of water. Bring the water to a boil over high heat.

2. Place the trimmed green beans in a steamer basket or colander that fits inside the saucepan. Make sure the water doesn't touch the bottom of the steamer.

3. Cover the saucepan with a lid and steam the green beans for 5•7 minutes, until they are tender•crisp. The green beans should be bright green and easily pierced with a fork.

4. Carefully remove the steamer basket or colander from the saucepan. Transfer the steamed green beans to a serving bowl.

5. If desired, season the green beans with a pinch of salt and black pepper.

6. Serve the steamed green beans warm.

Tips:
• For extra flavor, you can drizzle the green beans with a bit of lemon juice or low•sodium soy sauce.
• Avoid overcooking the green beans, as they can become mushy.
• Steaming is a great cooking method for gastric bypass patients as it preserves the nutrients and is gentle on the digestive system.

Steamed green beans are a simple, healthy, and easy•to•digest side dish that's perfect for a gastric bypass diet. The bright green color and tender•crisp texture make them a delicious and nutritious addition to any meal.

47. Spaghetti squash with tomato sauce

Ingredient:

- 1 medium spaghetti squash (about 3 lbs)
- 1 tablespoon olive oil
- 1 (14.5 oz) can diced tomatoes, no salt added
- 2 cloves garlic, minced
- 1 teaspoon dried oregano
- 1/4 teaspoon salt
- 1/8 teaspoon black pepper
- 2 tablespoons grated Parmesan cheese (optional)
- Fresh basil leaves for garnish (optional)

Instructions:

1. Preheat your oven to 400°F (200°C).

2. Cut the spaghetti squash in half lengthwise and scoop out the seeds. Place the squash halves cut·side up on a baking sheet.

3. Bake the spaghetti squash for 40·50 minutes, until tender when pierced with a fork.

4. While the squash is baking, in a small saucepan, heat the olive oil over medium heat. Add the minced garlic and sauté for 1 minute until fragrant.

5. Add the diced tomatoes, oregano, salt, and black pepper. Simmer the tomato sauce for 5·7 minutes, stirring occasionally.

6. Remove the baked spaghetti squash from the oven and let it cool for 5 minutes. Use a fork to gently scrape the flesh of the squash, separating it into spaghetti·like strands.

7. Transfer the spaghetti squash strands to a serving bowl. Top with the warm tomato sauce and grated Parmesan cheese, if using.

8. Garnish with fresh basil leaves, if desired.

9. Serve the spaghetti squash with tomato sauce warm.

Spaghetti squash is a low·carb, high·fiber alternative to traditional pasta, making it a great option for a gastric bypass diet. The tomato sauce provides a flavorful and nutrient·dense topping.

48. Roasted carrots

Ingredient:

- 1 lb carrots, peeled and cut into 1·inch pieces
- 1 tablespoon olive oil
- 1/4 teaspoon salt
- 1/8 teaspoon black pepper

Instructions:

1. Preheat your oven to 400°F (200°C).

2. In a large bowl, toss the peeled and cut carrots with the olive oil, salt, and black pepper until the carrots are evenly coated.

3. Spread the seasoned carrots in a single layer on a large baking sheet or rimmed baking dish.

4. Roast the carrots in the preheated oven for 20·25 minutes, tossing halfway through, until they are tender and lightly browned.

5. Remove the roasted carrots from the oven and transfer them to a serving dish.

Tips:
- For even cooking, try to cut the carrots into similar·sized pieces.
- You can also add other seasonings, such as garlic powder, cumin, or a sprinkle of Parmesan cheese.
- Roasting brings out the natural sweetness of the carrots and makes them deliciously tender.
- Roasted carrots can be served as a side dish or incorporated into other recipes, such as salads or grain bowls.

Carrots are an excellent source of fiber, vitamins, and minerals, making them a great choice for a gastric bypass diet. The roasting process makes them easy to digest and full of flavor.

49. Grilled eggplant

Ingredient:

• 1 medium eggplant, sliced into 1/2•inch thick rounds
• 1 tablespoon olive oil
• 1/4 teaspoon salt
• 1/8 teaspoon black pepper

Instructions:

1. Preheat your grill or grill pan to medium•high heat.

2. In a large bowl, toss the eggplant slices with the olive oil, salt, and black pepper until the eggplant is evenly coated.

3. Arrange the seasoned eggplant slices in a single layer on the preheated grill or grill pan.

4. Grill the eggplant for 3•4 minutes per side, or until tender and lightly charred.

5. Use tongs to transfer the grilled eggplant slices to a serving plate.

Tips:
• For best results, choose firm, fresh eggplant that is free of blemishes.
• You can also brush the eggplant slices with a bit of lemon juice or balsamic vinegar for extra flavor.
• Grilling brings out the natural sweetness of the eggplant and gives it a delicious smoky flavor.
• Grilled eggplant can be served as a side dish or incorporated into other recipes, such as salads or sandwiches.

Eggplant is a low•calorie, high•fiber vegetable that's rich in antioxidants. The grilling process makes it tender and easy to digest, making it a great choice for a gastric bypass diet.

50. Baked kale chips

Ingredient:

- 1 bunch of kale, stems removed and leaves torn into bite•sized pieces (about 4 cups)
- 1 tablespoon olive oil
- 1/4 teaspoon salt

Instructions:

1. Preheat your oven to 350°F (175°C).

2. Wash and thoroughly dry the kale leaves. Tear the leaves into bite•sized pieces, discarding the tough stems.

3. In a large bowl, toss the kale pieces with the olive oil and salt until the kale is evenly coated.

4. Spread the seasoned kale leaves in a single layer on a large baking sheet or two smaller baking sheets, making sure the leaves don't overlap.

5. Bake the kale chips in the preheated oven for 12•15 minutes, flipping the leaves halfway through, until they are crispy and lightly browned.

6. Remove the baked kale chips from the oven and let them cool for a few minutes before serving.

Tips:
- For extra flavor, you can sprinkle the kale chips with other seasonings like garlic powder, paprika, or Parmesan cheese.
- Make sure to thoroughly dry the kale leaves before baking to ensure they get crispy.
- Keep a close eye on the kale chips towards the end of the baking time to prevent them from burning.
- Baked kale chips are best enjoyed immediately, as they can lose their crispness over time.

Kale is an incredibly nutrient•dense leafy green that's high in fiber, vitamins, and minerals. Baking the kale into crispy chips makes for a satisfying and healthy snack option for a gastric bypass diet.

51. Roasted beets

Ingredient:

- 1 lb beets, peeled and cut into 1·inch cubes
- 1 tablespoon olive oil
- 1/4 teaspoon salt
- 1/8 teaspoon black pepper

Instructions:

1. Preheat your oven to 400°F (200°C).

2. In a large bowl, toss the cubed beets with the olive oil, salt, and black pepper until the beets are evenly coated.

3. Spread the seasoned beet cubes in a single layer on a large baking sheet or rimmed baking dish.

4. Roast the beets in the preheated oven for 25·30 minutes, tossing halfway through, until they are tender and lightly browned.

5. Remove the roasted beets from the oven and transfer them to a serving dish.

Tips:
- For even cooking, try to cut the beets into similar·sized cubes.
- You can also add other seasonings, such as garlic powder, thyme, or a sprinkle of Parmesan cheese.
- Roasting brings out the natural sweetness of the beets and makes them deliciously tender.
- Roasted beets can be served as a side dish or incorporated into other recipes, such as salads or grain bowls.

Beets are an excellent source of fiber, vitamins, and minerals, making them a great choice for a gastric bypass diet. The roasting process makes them easy to digest and full of flavor.

52. Steamed artichokes

Ingredient:

- 2 medium artichokes
- 1 lemon, cut in half
- 1/4 cup water
- 1/4 teaspoon salt

Instructions:

1. Prepare the artichokes:
   - Trim the stem of each artichoke, leaving about 1 inch.
   - Use kitchen shears to snip off the pointed tips of the artichoke leaves.
   - Rub the cut surfaces with the lemon halves to prevent browning.

2. In a large pot with a steamer basket, bring the water to a boil over high heat.

3. Place the prepared artichokes, stem•side down, in the steamer basket. Cover the pot with a lid.

4. Steam the artichokes for 25•35 minutes, until the leaves pull off easily and the base is tender when pierced with a fork.

5. Remove the steamed artichokes from the pot and transfer them to a serving plate. Sprinkle with the salt.

6. Serve the artichokes warm, with the lemon halves for squeezing over the leaves.

Tips:
• To eat, pull off the leaves one by one and scrape the tender, fleshy part at the base of each leaf with your teeth.
• The heart and stem of the artichoke are also edible and can be enjoyed.
• Steaming is a great cooking method for artichokes as it preserves their nutrients and makes them easy to digest.
• Artichokes are a good source of fiber, vitamins, and antioxidants, making them a great choice for a gastric bypass diet.

Enjoy these delicious and nutritious steamed artichokes as a side dish or appetizer!

53. Grilled portobello mushrooms

Ingredient:

- 4 large portobello mushroom caps, stems removed
- 2 tablespoons olive oil
- 1 tablespoon balsamic vinegar
- 2 cloves garlic, minced
- 1/4 teaspoon salt
- 1/8 teaspoon black pepper

Instructions:

1. Preheat your grill or grill pan to medium·high heat.

2. In a shallow dish, whisk together the olive oil, balsamic vinegar, minced garlic, salt, and black pepper.

3. Add the portobello mushroom caps to the dish and turn to coat them evenly with the marinade.

4. Place the marinated portobello caps directly on the preheated grill or grill pan, gill·side down.

5. Grill the mushrooms for 4·5 minutes per side, or until they are tender and lightly charred.

6. Use tongs to transfer the grilled portobello mushrooms to a serving plate.

Tips:
- For best results, choose fresh, firm portobello mushrooms that are free of blemishes.
- You can also marinate the mushrooms for 30 minutes to 1 hour before grilling to enhance the flavor.
- Grilling brings out the natural umami flavor of the portobello mushrooms and gives them a delicious smoky char.
- Grilled portobello mushrooms can be served as a side dish or used as a meat alternative in various recipes.

Portobello mushrooms are a great source of fiber, vitamins, and minerals, making them a healthy and satisfying option for a gastric bypass diet. The grilling process makes them tender and easy to digest.

54. Roasted butternut squash

Ingredient:

- 1 medium butternut squash, peeled, seeded, and cut into 1·inch cubes (about 4 cups)
- 1 tablespoon olive oil
- 1/2 teaspoon ground cinnamon
- 1/4 teaspoon ground nutmeg
- 1/4 teaspoon salt
- 1/8 teaspoon black pepper

Instructions:

1. Preheat your oven to 400°F (200°C).

2. In a large bowl, toss the cubed butternut squash with the olive oil, cinnamon, nutmeg, salt, and black pepper until the squash is evenly coated.

3. Spread the seasoned butternut squash in a single layer on a large baking sheet or rimmed baking dish.

4. Roast the butternut squash in the preheated oven for 25·30 minutes, tossing halfway through, until the squash is tender and lightly browned.

5. Remove the roasted butternut squash from the oven and transfer it to a serving dish.

Tips:
- For even cooking, try to cut the butternut squash into similar·sized cubes.
- You can also add other seasonings, such as garlic powder, paprika, or a sprinkle of Parmesan cheese.
- Roasting brings out the natural sweetness of the butternut squash and makes it deliciously tender.
- Roasted butternut squash can be served as a side dish or incorporated into other recipes, such as salads or grain bowls.

Butternut squash is an excellent source of fiber, vitamins, and minerals, making it a great choice for a gastric bypass diet. The roasting process makes it easy to digest and full of flavor.

55. Cauliflower rice

Ingredient:

- 1 pint cherry tomatoes, halved
- 1 tablespoon olive oil
- 2 cloves garlic, minced
- 1/4 teaspoon salt
- 1/8 teaspoon black pepper
- 2 tablespoons chopped fresh basil (optional)

Instructions:

1. In a large skillet, heat the olive oil over medium heat.

2. Add the halved cherry tomatoes and minced garlic to the skillet. Sauté for 5·7 minutes, stirring occasionally, until the tomatoes start to soften and release their juices.

3. Season the sautéed tomatoes with salt and black pepper. Stir to combine.

4. Remove the skillet from the heat and stir in the chopped fresh basil, if using.

5. Serve the sautéed cherry tomatoes warm, as a side dish or topping for other dishes.

Tips:
- For best flavor, use ripe, in·season cherry tomatoes.
- You can also add a splash of balsamic vinegar or a sprinkle of Parmesan cheese for extra flavor.
- Sautéing the tomatoes helps to concentrate their natural sweetness and brings out their vibrant color.
- Sautéed cherry tomatoes are a great way to incorporate more vegetables into your gastric bypass diet.

This simple sautéed cherry tomato dish is a delicious and nutritious side that's easy to digest. The bright, fresh flavors make it a great accompaniment to a variety of main dishes.

56. Sautéed cherry tomatoes

Ingredient:

- 1 pint cherry tomatoes, halved
- 1 tablespoon olive oil
- 2 cloves garlic, minced
- 1/4 teaspoon salt
- 1/8 teaspoon black pepper
- 2 tablespoons chopped fresh basil (optional)

Instructions:

1. In a large skillet, heat the olive oil over medium heat.

2. Add the halved cherry tomatoes and minced garlic to the skillet. Sauté for 5·7 minutes, stirring occasionally, until the tomatoes start to soften and release their juices.

3. Season the sautéed tomatoes with salt and black pepper. Stir to combine.

4. Remove the skillet from the heat and stir in the chopped fresh basil, if using.

5. Serve the sautéed cherry tomatoes warm, as a side dish or topping for other dishes.

Tips:
- For best flavor, use ripe, in·season cherry tomatoes.
- You can also add a splash of balsamic vinegar or a sprinkle of Parmesan cheese for extra flavor.
- Sautéing the tomatoes helps to concentrate their natural sweetness and brings out their vibrant color.
- Sautéed cherry tomatoes are a great way to incorporate more vegetables into your gastric bypass diet.

This simple sautéed cherry tomato dish is a delicious and nutritious side that's easy to digest. The bright, fresh flavors make it a great accompaniment to a variety of main dishes.

57. Steamed sugar snap peas

Ingredient:

• 1 lb sugar snap peas, trimmed
• 1•2 tablespoons water
• 1/4 teaspoon salt (optional)

Instructions:

1. In a medium saucepan, bring 1•2 tablespoons of water to a boil over high heat.

2. Add the trimmed sugar snap peas to the saucepan. Cover with a lid and steam the peas for 3•5 minutes, until they are tender•crisp.

3. Carefully remove the steamed sugar snap peas from the saucepan and transfer them to a serving bowl.

4. If desired, sprinkle the steamed peas with a pinch of salt.

5. Serve the steamed sugar snap peas warm.

Tips:
• For extra flavor, you can drizzle the steamed peas with a bit of lemon juice or low•sodium soy sauce.
• Avoid overcooking the sugar snap peas, as they can become mushy.
• Steaming is a great cooking method for gastric bypass patients as it preserves the nutrients and is gentle on the digestive system.

Sugar snap peas are a low•calorie, high•fiber vegetable that's rich in vitamins and minerals. The steaming process makes them tender and easy to digest, making them a great choice for a gastric bypass diet.

58. Roasted fennel

Ingredient:

- 2 medium fennel bulbs, trimmed and cut into 1/2·inch thick slices
- 1 tablespoon olive oil
- 1/4 teaspoon salt
- 1/8 teaspoon black pepper

Instructions:

1. Preheat your oven to 400°F (200°C).

2. In a large bowl, toss the sliced fennel with the olive oil, salt, and black pepper until the fennel is evenly coated.

3. Spread the seasoned fennel slices in a single layer on a large baking sheet or rimmed baking dish.

4. Roast the fennel in the preheated oven for 20·25 minutes, flipping the slices halfway through, until the fennel is tender and lightly browned.

5. Remove the roasted fennel from the oven and transfer it to a serving dish.

Tips:
- For even cooking, try to cut the fennel slices into similar thicknesses.
- You can also add other seasonings, such as garlic powder, lemon zest, or a sprinkle of Parmesan cheese.
- Roasting brings out the natural sweetness and anise·like flavor of the fennel.
- Roasted fennel can be served as a side dish or incorporated into other recipes, such as salads or grain bowls.

Fennel is a low·calorie, high·fiber vegetable that's rich in vitamins and minerals. The roasting process makes it tender and easy to digest, making it a great choice for a gastric bypass diet.

59. Grilled corn on the cob (without butter)

Ingredient:

- 4 ears of fresh corn, husks and silk removed
- 1 tablespoon olive oil
- 1/4 teaspoon salt
- 1/8 teaspoon black pepper

Instructions:

1. Preheat your grill or grill pan to medium·high heat.

2. In a large bowl, brush the corn cobs with the olive oil and sprinkle with the salt and black pepper, making sure to coat them evenly.

3. Place the seasoned corn cobs directly on the preheated grill or grill pan.

4. Grill the corn, turning occasionally, for 15·20 minutes, or until the kernels are tender and lightly charred.

5. Use tongs to transfer the grilled corn on the cob to a serving platter.

Tips:
- For extra flavor, you can rub the corn with a bit of garlic powder or chili powder before grilling.
- Grilling the corn adds a delicious smoky flavor without the need for butter or other high·fat toppings.
- Serve the grilled corn on the cob warm, and let your guests add any desired low·calorie toppings, such as a squeeze of lemon or a sprinkle of grated Parmesan cheese.

Corn on the cob is a tasty and versatile side dish that's perfect for a gastric bypass diet. The grilling process makes it tender and easy to digest, while keeping it low in calories and fat.

60. Baked acorn squash

Ingredient:

- 1 acorn squash, halved and seeded
- 2 tbsp butter or olive oil
- Salt and pepper to taste

Instructions:

1. Preheat the oven to 400°F (200°C).

2. Cut the acorn squash in half lengthwise and scoop out the seeds.

3. Place the squash halves cut•side up on a baking sheet.

4. Dot each half with 1 tbsp of butter or drizzle with 1 tbsp of olive oil. Season with salt and pepper.

5. Bake for 40•50 minutes, until the squash is very soft when pierced with a fork.

6. Serve the baked acorn squash halves as a side dish. You can scoop out the flesh and mash it if desired.

The natural sweetness of the acorn squash pairs beautifully with the butter or olive oil. This is a simple and delicious way to enjoy this fall vegetable.

61. Steamed edamame

Ingredient:

- 1 lb fresh edamame in the pod
- 1•2 tsp coarse sea salt or kosher salt

Instructions:

1. Bring a large pot of water to a boil.

2. Add the edamame pods to the boiling water. Cover and steam for 5•7 minutes, until the pods are bright green and tender.

3. Drain the edamame and transfer to a serving bowl.

4. Sprinkle the hot edamame generously with the coarse salt.

5. Serve the steamed edamame warm, with small bowls for the empty pods.

To eat, simply pick up an edamame pod, place it in your mouth, and use your teeth to gently squeeze the beans out of the pod. Discard the empty pod.

Edamame is a popular appetizer or snack, especially in Japanese cuisine. The salty, savory flavor pairs perfectly with the tender, slightly sweet beans. Steaming is the easiest way to prepare fresh edamame. Enjoy!

62. Roasted radishes

Ingredient:

- 1 lb radishes, trimmed and halved or quartered (depending on size)
- 1 tablespoon olive oil
- 1/4 teaspoon salt
- 1/8 teaspoon black pepper

Instructions:

1. Preheat your oven to 400°F (200°C).

2. In a large bowl, toss the trimmed and halved/quartered radishes with the olive oil, salt, and black pepper until the radishes are evenly coated.

3. Spread the seasoned radishes in a single layer on a large baking sheet or rimmed baking dish.

4. Roast the radishes in the preheated oven for 20•25 minutes, tossing halfway through, until they are tender and lightly browned.

5. Remove the roasted radishes from the oven and transfer them to a serving dish.

Tips:
- For even cooking, try to cut the radishes into similar•sized pieces.
- You can also add other seasonings, such as garlic powder, dried herbs, or a sprinkle of Parmesan cheese.
- Roasting brings out the natural sweetness of the radishes and makes them deliciously tender.
- Roasted radishes can be served as a side dish or incorporated into other recipes, such as salads or grain bowls.

Radishes are a low•calorie, high•fiber vegetable that's rich in vitamins and minerals. The roasting process makes them easy to digest and full of flavor, making them a great choice for a gastric bypass diet.

63. Sautéed mushrooms

Ingredient:

- 1 lb mushrooms, sliced (such as cremini, button, or shiitake)
- 2 tbsp butter or olive oil
- 2 cloves garlic, minced
- 1 tbsp fresh thyme leaves (or 1 tsp dried thyme)
- Salt and pepper to taste

Instructions:

1. Clean the mushrooms by wiping them with a damp paper towel to remove any dirt or debris. Slice the mushrooms.

2. In a large skillet or sauté pan, melt the butter (or heat the olive oil) over medium•high heat.

3. Add the sliced mushrooms in a single layer and let them cook undisturbed for 2•3 minutes to allow them to brown on the bottom.

4. Stir the mushrooms and continue cooking for 5•7 minutes, stirring occasionally, until they are tender and lightly browned.

5. Add the minced garlic and thyme. Cook for 1 minute more, stirring constantly, until fragrant.

6. Season the sautéed mushrooms with salt and pepper to taste.

7. Serve the sautéed mushrooms warm, as a side dish or topping for steaks, burgers, pasta, etc.

The key to getting nicely browned, flavorful mushrooms is to not overcrowd the pan and let them sear properly before stirring. Adjust the cooking time as needed based on the type and size of your mushrooms. Enjoy!

64. Grilled red bell peppers

Ingredient:

- 4 large red bell peppers
- Olive oil
- Salt and pepper

Instructions:

1. Preheat your grill to medium•high heat.

2. Wash the red bell peppers and pat them dry. Brush or drizzle them lightly with olive oil and season with salt and pepper.

3. Place the peppers directly on the grill grates. Grill for 12•15 minutes, turning occasionally, until the skins are charred and blistered on all sides.

4. Transfer the grilled peppers to a bowl and cover with plastic wrap or a lid. Let them steam for 10•15 minutes. This will make the skins easier to peel.

5. Remove the peppers from the bowl. Peel off the charred skins, leaving the peppers intact. You can also remove the stems and seeds if desired.

6. Slice the grilled red peppers into strips or leave them whole. Drizzle with a bit more olive oil if desired.

The grilled red peppers can be served as a side dish, added to salads, sandwiches, or used in other recipes. The smoky, charred flavor is delicious. Enjoy!

65. Roasted turnips

Ingredient:

- 1 lb turnips, peeled and cut into 1·inch cubes
- 2 tbsp olive oil
- 1 tsp dried thyme
- Salt and pepper to taste

Instructions:

1. Preheat your oven to 400°F (200°C).

2. In a large bowl, toss the cubed turnips with the olive oil, dried thyme, and a generous pinch of salt and pepper.

3. Spread the seasoned turnips in a single layer on a baking sheet lined with parchment paper.

4. Roast the turnips for 25·30 minutes, flipping halfway, until they are tender and lightly browned.

5. Remove the roasted turnips from the oven and transfer to a serving dish.

6. Taste and adjust seasoning with additional salt and pepper if desired.

The roasting process brings out the natural sweetness of the turnips and gives them a nice caramelized exterior. Turnips are a versatile root vegetable that pair well with herbs and spices.

You can also try adding other vegetables like carrots, potatoes, or onions to the roasting pan. Roasted turnips make a great side dish or can be added to soups, stews, or salads.

66. Steamed bok choy

Ingredient:

- 1 lb baby bok choy, rinsed and trimmed
- 1 tbsp sesame oil
- 1 tbsp soy sauce
- 1 tsp rice vinegar
- 1 tsp toasted sesame seeds (optional)
- Salt and pepper to taste

Instructions:

1. Bring a large pot of water to a boil. Set up a steamer basket or colander over the pot.

2. Add the trimmed bok choy to the steamer basket. Cover and steam for 5·7 minutes, until the bok choy is tender but still crisp.

3. Transfer the steamed bok choy to a serving bowl.

4. In a small bowl, whisk together the sesame oil, soy sauce, and rice vinegar.

5. Drizzle the sesame dressing over the hot bok choy and toss gently to coat.

6. Sprinkle the bok choy with toasted sesame seeds, if using. Season with salt and pepper to taste.

7. Serve the steamed bok choy warm or at room temperature.

The tender, slightly sweet bok choy pairs beautifully with the savory sesame dressing. Steaming is a quick and healthy way to prepare this Chinese green vegetable. Adjust the cooking time as needed based on the size of your bok choy pieces.

67. Grilled asparagus with lemon

Ingredient:

- 1 lb asparagus, woody ends trimmed
- 2 tbsp olive oil
- 1 tbsp lemon juice
- 1 tsp lemon zest
- Salt and pepper to taste

Instructions:

1. Preheat your grill to medium•high heat.

2. In a large bowl, toss the asparagus spears with the olive oil, lemon juice, and a pinch of salt and pepper.

3. Arrange the asparagus in a single layer on the hot grill grates. Grill for 5•7 minutes, turning occasionally, until the asparagus is tender•crisp and lightly charred.

4. Transfer the grilled asparagus to a serving platter. Sprinkle with the lemon zest and additional salt and pepper to taste.

5. Serve the grilled asparagus warm or at room temperature.

The high heat of the grill brings out the natural sweetness of the asparagus and gives it a nice smoky flavor. The lemon juice and zest provide a bright, refreshing contrast.

You can also try adding other seasonings like garlic powder, red pepper flakes, or Parmesan cheese to the asparagus before grilling. Grilled asparagus makes a great side dish or can be added to salads, pasta, or grain bowls.

68. Roasted parsnips

Ingredient:

• 1 lb parsnips, peeled and cut into 1•inch pieces
• 2 tbsp olive oil
• 1 tsp dried thyme
• 1 tsp paprika
• Salt and pepper to taste

Instructions:

1. Preheat your oven to 400°F (200°C).

2. In a large bowl, toss the parsnip pieces with the olive oil, dried thyme, paprika, and a generous pinch of salt and pepper.

3. Spread the seasoned parsnips in a single layer on a baking sheet lined with parchment paper.

4. Roast the parsnips for 25•30 minutes, flipping halfway, until they are tender and lightly browned.

5. Remove the roasted parsnips from the oven and transfer to a serving dish.

6. Taste and adjust seasoning with additional salt and pepper if desired.

The key to getting nicely roasted parsnips is to cut them into evenly sized pieces so they cook through at the same rate. The thyme and paprika add great flavor, but you can also experiment with other spices like garlic powder, cumin, or rosemary.

Roasted parsnips make a delicious side dish, but you can also toss them into salads, soups, or stews. They have a sweet, earthy flavor that pairs well with many different meals.

69. Sautéed Swiss chard

Ingredient:

• 1 bunch Swiss chard, stems removed and leaves chopped
• 1 tbsp olive oil
• 2 cloves garlic, minced
• 1/4 cup low•sodium vegetable or chicken broth
• 1 tsp lemon juice
• Salt and pepper to taste

Instructions:

1. Heat the olive oil in a large skillet or sauté pan over medium heat.

2. Add the minced garlic and sauté for 1 minute, until fragrant.

3. Add the chopped Swiss chard leaves to the pan and sauté for 2•3 minutes, until the leaves start to wilt.

4. Pour in the low•sodium broth and lemon juice. Stir to combine.

5. Cover the pan and let the chard simmer for 5•7 minutes, or until the leaves are tender.

6. Remove the lid and continue cooking for 1•2 minutes to allow any excess liquid to evaporate.

7. Season the sautéed Swiss chard with salt and pepper to taste.

8. Serve the chard warm.

Tips:
• Swiss chard is a nutrient•dense leafy green that is easy to digest after gastric bypass surgery.
• The sautéing method helps soften the chard and make it more palatable.
• The lemon juice and garlic add flavor without the need for high•fat seasonings or sauces.
• Serve the sautéed Swiss chard as a side dish or incorporate it into other gastric bypass•friendly meals.
• Be sure to chew the chard thoroughly and eat slowly to prevent discomfort.

70. Baked rutabaga fries

Ingredient:

- 1 lb rutabaga, peeled and cut into 1/2•inch thick fry shapes
- 2 tbsp olive oil
- 1 tsp garlic powder
- 1 tsp paprika
- 1/2 tsp salt
- 1/4 tsp black pepper

Instructions:

1. Preheat your oven to 400°F (200°C). Line a baking sheet with parchment paper.

2. In a large bowl, toss the cut rutabaga fries with the olive oil, garlic powder, paprika, salt, and pepper until evenly coated.

3. Spread the seasoned rutabaga fries in a single layer on the prepared baking sheet.

4. Bake for 25•30 minutes, flipping halfway, until the fries are tender and lightly browned.

5. Remove the baked rutabaga fries from the oven and transfer to a serving dish.

6. Serve the rutabaga fries hot, garnished with additional salt and pepper if desired.

The key to getting crispy baked rutabaga fries is to cut them into even, thin pieces and make sure they are in a single layer on the baking sheet. The high heat and flipping helps them get nicely browned.

Rutabagas have a slightly sweet, earthy flavor that pairs well with the garlic and paprika seasoning. You can also experiment with other spice blends like cajun, Italian, or ranch seasoning.

71. Fresh berries

Ingredient:

- 1 lb mixed fresh berries (such as strawberries, blueberries, raspberries, blackberries)
- 1•2 tbsp granulated sugar (optional)
- Fresh mint leaves (optional)

Instructions:

1. Rinse the fresh berries gently under cool running water. Pat them dry with paper towels or a clean kitchen towel.

2. Transfer the berries to a serving bowl or plate.

3. If desired, sprinkle the berries lightly with granulated sugar. This will help bring out their natural sweetness.

4. Garnish the fresh berries with a few fresh mint leaves, if desired.

5. Serve the fresh berries immediately, or refrigerate until ready to serve.

That's it! Fresh, ripe berries are a simple and delicious treat on their own. You can also use them in a variety of ways:

- Top them on yogurt, oatmeal, or cereal
- Fold them into whipped cream or mascarpone for a quick dessert
- Make a mixed berry salad with a light drizzle of honey or balsamic glaze
- Blend them into smoothies or use them in baked goods like pies, cobblers, or muffins

The key is to use the freshest, ripest berries you can find. Enjoy the natural sweetness and vibrant colors of this seasonal fruit!

72. Apple slices with almond butter

Ingredient:

- 1•2 apples, cored and sliced
- 2•3 tablespoons creamy or crunchy almond butter

Instructions:

1. Wash and core the apples. Slice them into thin wedges or rounds.

2. Arrange the apple slices on a plate or platter.

3. Scoop the almond butter into a small bowl or ramekin.

4. Serve the apple slices alongside the almond butter for dipping.

That's it! This is a simple, nutritious snack that combines the sweetness of fresh apples with the protein and healthy fats from the almond butter.

Some variations and tips:

- Use any type of apple you prefer • Gala, Honeycrisp, Fuji, etc.

- For extra flavor, you can sprinkle the apple slices with a bit of cinnamon.

- Try using other nut butters like peanut butter or cashew butter.

- Add a drizzle of honey or maple syrup to the almond butter if desired.

- Sprinkle the almond butter with chopped nuts, seeds, or granola for extra crunch.

This makes a great snack or light dessert. The combination of crisp apples and creamy, nutty almond butter is both satisfying and delicious. Enjoy!

73. Carrot sticks with hummus

Ingredient:

• 4•5 medium carrots, peeled and cut into sticks
• 1/2 cup hummus (store•bought or homemade)

Instructions:

1. Wash and peel the carrots. Cut them into long, thin sticks, about 4•5 inches long.

2. Arrange the carrot sticks on a plate or in a shallow bowl.

3. Scoop the hummus into a small bowl or ramekin and place it next to the carrot sticks.

That's it! This makes a simple, nutritious snack.

The crunchy, sweet carrot sticks pair perfectly with the creamy, savory hummus. Hummus is a great source of plant•based protein, fiber, and healthy fats from the chickpeas and tahini.

Some variations and tips:

• Try different flavors of hummus like roasted red pepper, garlic, or Mediterranean.

• Add a sprinkle of paprika, za'atar, or chopped fresh herbs on top of the hummus.

• For extra flavor, you can drizzle a bit of olive oil over the hummus.

• Serve the carrot sticks and hummus with other fresh veggies like celery, cucumber, or bell pepper strips.

• This makes a great healthy snack or appetizer for parties and gatherings.

The combination of crunchy carrots and creamy hummus is both satisfying and delicious. Enjoy!

74. Cucumber slices with low•fat cream cheese

Ingredient:

• 1 medium cucumber, washed and sliced into rounds
• 4 oz low•fat or reduced•fat cream cheese, softened

Instructions:

1. Wash the cucumber and slice it into rounds, about 1/4•inch thick.

2. Spread a small amount of the softened cream cheese onto each cucumber slice.

3. Arrange the cucumber slices with cream cheese on a plate or platter.

That's it! This makes a refreshing and nutritious snack.

The cool, crisp cucumber pairs perfectly with the creamy, tangy cream cheese. It's a simple but delicious combination.

Some variations and tips:

• Try using different flavors of cream cheese, like chive, garlic, or herb.

• For extra flavor, you can sprinkle the cucumber slices with a bit of salt, pepper, or dried herbs before adding the cream cheese.

• You can also top the cream cheese with a small piece of fresh dill, chives, or a sprinkle of paprika.

• Serve the cucumber slices with cream cheese as part of a veggie tray or appetizer platter.

• For a heartier snack, you can add a small slice of smoked salmon or a sprinkle of chopped nuts on top of the cream cheese.

This makes a refreshing, low•calorie snack that's high in fiber, vitamins, and protein from the cream cheese. Enjoy!

75. Celery sticks with low•fat peanut butter

Ingredient:

• 3•4 celery stalks, washed and cut into 4•inch sticks
• 2•3 tablespoons low•fat or reduced•fat peanut butter

Instructions:

1. Wash the celery stalks and cut them into 4•inch sticks.

2. Spread a small amount of the peanut butter onto each celery stick.

3. Arrange the celery sticks with peanut butter on a plate or platter.

That's it! This makes a simple, nutritious, and satisfying snack.

The crunchy celery sticks provide a nice contrast to the creamy, nutty peanut butter. It's a great combination of fiber, protein, and healthy fats.

Some variations and tips:

• Try using different nut or seed butters like almond butter, cashew butter, or sunflower seed butter.

• For extra flavor, you can sprinkle the peanut butter•topped celery sticks with a pinch of cinnamon, cocoa powder, or chopped nuts.

• Add a drizzle of honey or maple syrup to the peanut butter for a touch of sweetness.

• Serve the celery sticks with peanut butter as part of a veggie tray or alongside other healthy snacks.

• For a heartier snack, you can top the peanut butter with raisins, dried cranberries, or mini chocolate chips.

This makes a great on•the•go snack that's high in fiber, vitamins, and protein. Enjoy!

76. Cherry tomatoes with low•fat mozzarella

Ingredient:

• 1 pint cherry or grape tomatoes, washed
• 4 oz low•fat or part•skim mozzarella cheese, cut into small cubes
• 1 tbsp balsamic glaze or reduction (optional)
• Fresh basil leaves, chopped (optional)
• Salt and pepper to taste

Instructions:

1. Wash the cherry tomatoes and pat them dry.

2. Cut the mozzarella cheese into small 1/2•inch cubes.

3. Arrange the cherry tomatoes and mozzarella cubes on a serving plate or platter.

4. Drizzle the balsamic glaze over the top, if using.

5. Sprinkle the chopped fresh basil over the top, if using.

6. Season with a pinch of salt and pepper.

That's it! This makes a simple, refreshing, and nutritious snack.

The juicy, sweet cherry tomatoes pair perfectly with the creamy, mild mozzarella cheese. The balsamic glaze and fresh basil add a nice flavor boost.

Some variations and tips:

• Try using different types of small tomatoes like grape, Sun Gold, or cherry.
• For extra protein, you can add a few slices of prosciutto or salami.
• Swap the mozzarella for small balls of burrata or fresh mozzarella.
• Drizzle a bit of high•quality olive oil over the top instead of balsamic.
• Sprinkle with a pinch of red pepper flakes for a little heat.
• Serve the tomato and mozzarella skewers as an appetizer or snack.

This makes a great healthy, low•calorie snack that's high in vitamins, minerals, and protein. Enjoy!

77. Watermelon cubes

Ingredient:

- 1 small watermelon, chilled
- Optional garnishes:
  - Fresh mint leaves
  - Lime wedges
  - Feta cheese crumbles
  - Balsamic glaze

Instructions:

1. Wash the watermelon and cut it in half lengthwise. Scoop out the seeds.

2. Cut the watermelon flesh into 1·inch cubes and transfer them to a serving bowl or platter.

3. Chill the watermelon cubes in the refrigerator for at least 30 minutes before serving.

4. When ready to serve, you can optionally garnish the watermelon cubes with:
   - Fresh mint leaves
   - Lime wedges for squeezing over the top
   - Crumbled feta cheese
   - A drizzle of balsamic glaze

That's it! Watermelon cubes make a refreshing, hydrating, and naturally sweet snack or dessert.

The chilled watermelon is perfect for hot summer days. The optional garnishes like mint, lime, feta, and balsamic can add extra flavor and contrast.

Tips:
- Choose a ripe, juicy watermelon for the best flavor.
- Chill the watermelon thoroughly before cutting and serving for maximum refreshment.
- Experiment with different flavor combinations · try adding a sprinkle of chili powder or a drizzle of honey.
- Watermelon cubes also make a great addition to fruit salads, smoothies, or cocktails.

78. Cantaloupe slices

Ingredient:

- 1 ripe cantaloupe
- Optional garnishes:
  - Lime wedges
  - Mint leaves
  - Honey or agave nectar
  - Chili powder or cayenne pepper

Instructions:

1. Wash the cantaloupe and slice it in half lengthwise. Scoop out the seeds.

2. Use a sharp knife to slice the cantaloupe flesh into half•moon or wedge shapes, about 1/2•inch thick.

3. Arrange the cantaloupe slices on a serving platter or plate.

4. If desired, you can garnish the cantaloupe slices with any of the following:
   - Lime wedges for squeezing over the top
   - Fresh mint leaves
   - A drizzle of honey or agave nectar
   - A light sprinkle of chili powder or cayenne pepper

That's it! Cantaloupe slices make a refreshing, hydrating, and naturally sweet snack or side dish.

The juicy, sweet cantaloupe is perfect for hot summer days. The optional garnishes can add extra flavor and contrast.

Tips:
- Choose a ripe, fragrant cantaloupe for the best flavor.
- Chill the cantaloupe thoroughly before slicing and serving for maximum refreshment.
- Experiment with different flavor combinations • try adding a sprinkle of lime zest or a pinch of salt.
- Cantaloupe slices also make a great addition to fruit salads, smoothies, or as a topping for yogurt or ice cream.

79. Honeydew melon balls

Ingredient:

• 1 ripe honeydew melon
• Optional garnishes:
  • Lime wedges
  • Fresh mint leaves
  • Honey or agave nectar
  • Toasted coconut flakes

Instructions:

1. Wash the honeydew melon and slice it in half lengthwise. Scoop out the seeds.

2. Use a melon baller or small spoon to scoop out round balls of the honeydew flesh.

3. Transfer the honeydew melon balls to a serving bowl or platter.

4. If desired, you can garnish the honeydew melon balls with any of the following:
  • Lime wedges for squeezing over the top
  • Fresh mint leaves
  • A drizzle of honey or agave nectar
  • A sprinkle of toasted coconut flakes

That's it! Honeydew melon balls make a refreshing, hydrating, and naturally sweet snack or side dish.

The juicy, sweet honeydew is perfect for hot summer days. The optional garnishes can add extra flavor and contrast.

Tips:
• Choose a ripe, fragrant honeydew for the best flavor.
• Chill the honeydew thoroughly before scooping and serving for maximum refreshment.
• Experiment with different flavor combinations • try adding a sprinkle of lime zest or a pinch of salt.
• Honeydew melon balls also make a great addition to fruit salads, smoothies, or as a topping for yogurt or ice cream.

80. Peach slices

Ingredient:

- 2•3 ripe peaches, pitted and sliced
- Optional toppings:
  - Honey or maple syrup
  - Chopped fresh mint or basil
  - Crumbled feta or ricotta cheese
  - Toasted sliced almonds or chopped walnuts
  - Squeeze of fresh lemon or lime juice

Instructions:

1. Wash the peaches and pat them dry. Cut each peach in half and remove the pit. Then slice the peach halves into 1/2•inch thick wedges.

2. Arrange the peach slices on a serving plate or platter.

3. If desired, you can drizzle the peach slices with a bit of honey or maple syrup to enhance their natural sweetness.

4. Top the peach slices with any of the optional toppings you'd like • fresh herbs, crumbled cheese, toasted nuts, or a squeeze of citrus.

That's it! The fresh, juicy peach slices make a simple and delicious snack or dessert.

Peaches have a wonderful sweet, aromatic flavor that pairs well with a variety of toppings. The optional garnishes can add extra flavor, texture, and nutrition.

You can also use the peach slices in salads, on top of yogurt or oatmeal, or as a topping for grilled meats or fish. They're a versatile fruit that work well in both sweet and savory dishes.

81. Nectarine wedges

Ingredient:

- 2•3 ripe nectarines, pitted and cut into wedges
- Optional toppings:
  - Honey or maple syrup
  - Chopped fresh mint or basil
  - Crumbled feta or ricotta cheese
  - Toasted nuts (such as almonds or pecans)
  - Squeeze of fresh lemon or lime juice

Instructions:

1. Wash the nectarines and pat them dry. Cut each nectarine in half and remove the pit. Then slice each half into 4•6 wedges.

2. Arrange the nectarine wedges on a serving plate or platter.

3. If desired, drizzle the nectarine wedges with a bit of honey or maple syrup to enhance their natural sweetness.

4. Top the nectarine wedges with any of the optional toppings you'd like • fresh herbs, crumbled cheese, toasted nuts, or a squeeze of citrus.

That's it! The fresh, juicy nectarine wedges make a simple and delicious snack or dessert.

You can also use the nectarine wedges in salads, on top of yogurt or oatmeal, or as a topping for grilled meats or fish. The sweet•tart flavor pairs well with savory and creamy elements.

82. Plum halves

Ingredient:

- 4•6 ripe plums, halved and pitted
- Optional toppings:
  - Honey or agave nectar
  - Chopped fresh mint or basil
  - Crumbled feta or goat cheese
  - Toasted sliced almonds or chopped walnuts
  - Squeeze of fresh lemon or lime juice

Instructions:

1. Wash the plums and pat them dry. Cut each plum in half and remove the pit.

2. Arrange the plum halves on a serving plate or platter.

3. If desired, you can drizzle the plum halves with a bit of honey or agave nectar to enhance their natural sweetness.

4. Top the plum halves with any of the optional toppings you'd like • fresh herbs, crumbled cheese, toasted nuts, or a squeeze of citrus.

That's it! The fresh, juicy plum halves make a simple and delicious snack or dessert.

Plums have a wonderful sweet•tart flavor that pairs well with a variety of toppings. The optional garnishes can add extra flavor, texture, and nutrition.

You can also use the plum halves in salads, on top of yogurt or oatmeal, or as a topping for grilled meats or fish. They're a versatile fruit that work well in both sweet and savory dishes.

83. Kiwi slices

Ingredient:

• 2•3 ripe kiwi fruits, peeled and sliced
• Optional toppings:
  • Honey or agave nectar
  • Chopped fresh mint or basil
  • Squeeze of fresh lime juice
  • Toasted coconut flakes or chopped nuts

Instructions:

1. Wash the kiwi fruits and peel off the fuzzy brown skin. Slice the kiwi into 1/4•inch thick rounds.

2. Arrange the kiwi slices on a serving plate or platter.

3. If desired, you can drizzle the kiwi slices with a bit of honey or agave nectar to enhance their natural sweetness.

4. Top the kiwi slices with any of the optional toppings you'd like • fresh herbs, a squeeze of lime juice, toasted coconut, or chopped nuts.

That's it! The bright green, juicy kiwi slices make a simple and refreshing snack or addition to fruit salads.

Kiwi has a sweet•tart flavor and is packed with vitamin C, fiber, and other beneficial nutrients. The optional garnishes can add extra flavor, texture, and visual appeal.

Tips:
• Choose ripe, soft kiwi fruits for the best flavor and texture.
• Slice the kiwi just before serving for maximum freshness.
• Experiment with different flavor combinations • try adding a pinch of chili powder or a drizzle of balsamic glaze.
• Kiwi slices also make a great topping for yogurt, oatmeal, or ice cream.

84. Pineapple chunks

Ingredient:

- 1 ripe pineapple, peeled, cored, and cut into 1·inch chunks
- Optional toppings:
  - Lime wedges
  - Chopped fresh mint or cilantro
  - Chili powder or cayenne pepper
  - Honey or agave nectar

Instructions:

1. Wash the pineapple and slice off the top and bottom. Use a sharp knife to peel off the tough outer skin, removing any remaining eyes or brown spots.

2. Cut the pineapple in half lengthwise, then slice each half into 1·inch thick slices. Cut the slices into 1·inch chunks.

3. Arrange the fresh pineapple chunks on a serving plate or platter.

4. If desired, you can top the pineapple chunks with any of the following:
   - Lime wedges for squeezing over the top
   - Chopped fresh mint or cilantro
   - A light sprinkle of chili powder or cayenne pepper
   - A drizzle of honey or agave nectar

That's it! Pineapple chunks make a refreshing, sweet, and juicy snack or addition to fruit salads.

The bright, tropical flavor of pineapple pairs well with the optional toppings. The lime, herbs, and spices can add a nice contrast to the natural sweetness.

Tips:
- Choose a ripe, fragrant pineapple for the best flavor.
- Chill the pineapple chunks in the refrigerator before serving for maximum refreshment.
- Experiment with different flavor combinations · try adding a sprinkle of toasted coconut or a drizzle of balsamic glaze.
- Pineapple chunks also make a great addition to smoothies, yogurt parfaits, or as a topping for grilled meats or fish.

85. Mango cubes

Ingredient:

• 2•3 ripe mangoes, peeled and cubed
• Optional toppings:
  • Lime wedges
  • Chopped fresh cilantro or mint
  • Chili powder or cayenne pepper
  • Honey or agave nectar

Instructions:

1. Wash the mangoes and use a sharp knife to peel off the skin. Cut the flesh away from the pit in long slices.

2. Dice the mango slices into 1•inch cubes.

3. Arrange the fresh mango cubes on a serving plate or platter.

4. If desired, you can top the mango cubes with any of the following:
  • Lime wedges for squeezing over the top
  • Chopped fresh cilantro or mint
  • A light sprinkle of chili powder or cayenne pepper
  • A drizzle of honey or agave nectar

That's it! Mango cubes make a refreshing, sweet, and juicy snack or addition to fruit salads.

The bright, tropical flavor of mango pairs well with the optional toppings. The lime, herbs, and spices can add a nice contrast to the natural sweetness.

Tips:
• Choose ripe, fragrant mangoes for the best flavor and texture.
• Chill the mango cubes in the refrigerator before serving for maximum refreshment.
• Experiment with different flavor combinations • try adding a sprinkle of toasted coconut or a drizzle of balsamic glaze.
• Mango cubes also make a great addition to smoothies, yogurt parfaits, or as a topping for grilled meats or fish.

86. Papaya slices

Ingredient:

- 1 ripe papaya, peeled, seeded, and sliced
- Optional toppings:
  - Lime wedges
  - Chopped fresh mint or cilantro
  - Pinch of chili powder or cayenne pepper (optional)

Instructions:

1. Wash the papaya and use a sharp knife to peel off the skin. Cut the papaya in half lengthwise and scoop out the seeds.

2. Slice the papaya flesh into 1/2•inch thick slices.

3. Arrange the fresh papaya slices on a serving plate or platter.

4. If desired, you can top the papaya slices with:
   - Lime wedges for squeezing over the top
   - Chopped fresh mint or cilantro
   - A light sprinkle of chili powder or cayenne pepper (for a touch of heat)

That's it! Papaya slices make a refreshing, sweet, and nutrient•dense snack that is well•suited for a gastric bypass diet.

Papaya is high in fiber, vitamins, and enzymes, making it easy to digest. The natural sweetness and juicy texture of the fruit can satisfy cravings without being too heavy.

Tips for a gastric bypass diet:
- Choose ripe, soft papaya for the best flavor and texture.
- Stick to small, 1/2•inch thick slices to prevent overeating.
- Avoid adding any heavy toppings or sauces that could be difficult to digest.
- Pair the papaya with other easy•to•digest foods like Greek yogurt or grilled chicken.
- Drink plenty of water before, during, and after eating to aid digestion.

87. Guava halves

Ingredient:

- 2•3 ripe guavas, halved
- Optional toppings:
  - Lime wedges
  - Chopped fresh cilantro or mint
  - Honey or agave nectar
  - Chili powder or cayenne pepper

Instructions:

1. Wash the guavas and cut them in half lengthwise. Leave the skin on.

2. Arrange the guava halves on a serving plate or platter.

3. If desired, you can top the guava halves with any of the following:
   - Lime wedges for squeezing over the top
   - Chopped fresh cilantro or mint
   - A drizzle of honey or agave nectar
   - A light sprinkle of chili powder or cayenne pepper

That's it! Guava halves make a refreshing, sweet, and tropical snack.

Guavas have a unique, slightly tart flavor that pairs well with the optional toppings. The lime, herbs, and spices can add a nice contrast to the natural sweetness of the fruit.

Tips:
- Choose ripe, fragrant guavas that are slightly soft to the touch.

- Chill the guava halves in the refrigerator before serving for maximum refreshment.

- Scoop out the soft, seedy interior of the guava halves with a spoon if desired.

- Experiment with different flavor combinations • try adding a sprinkle of toasted coconut or a drizzle of balsamic glaze.

- Guava halves also make a great addition to fruit salads or as a topping for yogurt or ice cream.

88. Passion fruit halves

Ingredient:

- 2•3 ripe passion fruits, halved
- Optional toppings:
  - Honey or agave nectar
  - Lime wedges
  - Chopped fresh mint or basil
  - Yogurt or whipped cream

Instructions:

1. Wash the passion fruits and cut them in half lengthwise.

2. Arrange the passion fruit halves on a serving plate or bowl.

3. If desired, you can top the passion fruit halves with any of the following:
   - A drizzle of honey or agave nectar to enhance the sweetness
   - Lime wedges for squeezing over the top
   - Chopped fresh mint or basil
   - A dollop of plain yogurt or whipped cream

That's it! Passion fruit halves make a refreshing, tangy, and tropical snack or dessert.

The bright, tart•sweet flavor of passion fruit is unique and delicious. The optional toppings can add extra sweetness, acidity, and creaminess to balance out the natural tartness.

Tips:
- Choose ripe passion fruits that are slightly wrinkled and give slightly when gently squeezed.
- Scoop out the soft, jelly•like pulp and seeds from the passion fruit halves with a spoon.
- Chill the passion fruit halves in the refrigerator before serving for maximum refreshment.
- Experiment with different flavor combinations • try adding a sprinkle of toasted coconut or a drizzle of balsamic glaze.
- Passion fruit halves also make a great addition to fruit salads, smoothies, or as a topping for yogurt or ice cream.

89. Pomegranate seeds

Ingredient:

- 1 pomegranate, seeded
- Optional toppings:
  - Squeeze of fresh lemon or lime juice
  - Chopped fresh mint or basil
  - Drizzle of honey or agave nectar
  - Sprinkle of ground cinnamon or cardamom

Instructions:

1. Cut the pomegranate in half and use your fingers to gently remove the seeds from the white membranes.

2. Transfer the pomegranate seeds to a serving bowl or plate.

3. If desired, you can top the pomegranate seeds with any of the following:
   - A squeeze of fresh lemon or lime juice
   - Chopped fresh mint or basil
   - A drizzle of honey or agave nectar
   - A sprinkle of ground cinnamon or cardamom

That's it! Pomegranate seeds make a refreshing, sweet•tart, and nutritious snack.

Pomegranate seeds are packed with antioxidants, fiber, and vitamins. They have a unique, juicy crunch that makes them a great addition to salads, yogurt, oatmeal, or even cocktails.

Tips:
- Choose a ripe pomegranate that feels heavy for its size and has a deep red color.
- Gently remove the seeds under water to prevent the juice from staining your hands.
- Chill the pomegranate seeds in the refrigerator before serving for a refreshing snack.
- Experiment with different flavor combinations • try adding a sprinkle of toasted nuts or a drizzle of balsamic glaze.

90. Grapefruit segments

Ingredient:

- 1·2 ruby red or pink grapefruits
- Optional toppings:
  - Honey or agave nectar
  - Mint leaves
  - Lime wedges

Instructions:

1. Slice the grapefruit in half horizontally. Use a sharp knife to carefully cut along the membranes to release the grapefruit segments.

2. Gently pull the grapefruit segments out of the rind and transfer them to a serving bowl or plate.

3. If desired, you can top the grapefruit segments with any of the following:
   - A drizzle of honey or agave nectar to balance the tartness
   - Chopped fresh mint leaves
   - Lime wedges for squeezing over the top

That's it! Grapefruit segments make a refreshing, tangy, and juicy snack.

The bright, citrusy flavor of grapefruit is a great way to start the day or enjoy as a light dessert. The optional toppings can add extra sweetness, acidity, and herbal notes.

Tips:

• Choose ripe, juicy grapefruits that are heavy for their size.

• Segment the grapefruit over a bowl to catch any dripping juice.

• Chill the grapefruit segments in the refrigerator before serving for maximum refreshment.

• Experiment with different varieties of grapefruit • try using a mix of red, pink, and white.

• Grapefruit segments also make a great addition to salads, yogurt parfaits, or as a topping for fish or poultry dishes.

91. Dates (in moderation)

Ingredient:

- 4•6 fresh Medjool or Deglet Noor dates
- Optional toppings:
  - Almond butter or peanut butter
  - Chopped nuts (such as almonds, walnuts, or pecans)
  - Shredded coconut
  - Cinnamon or cocoa powder

Instructions:

1. Wash the dates and pat them dry. Slice them in half lengthwise, or leave them whole if they are small.

2. Arrange the date halves or whole dates on a serving plate or platter.

3. If desired, you can top the dates with any of the following:
   - A small spoonful of almond butter or peanut butter
   - Chopped nuts like almonds, walnuts, or pecans
   - A sprinkle of shredded coconut
   - A light dusting of cinnamon or cocoa powder

That's it! Dates make a naturally sweet and satisfying snack, but they should be consumed in moderation due to their high sugar content.

Dates are a good source of fiber, vitamins, and minerals. The optional toppings can add extra protein, healthy fats, and flavor to balance out the sweetness.

Tips:
- Choose soft, plump Medjool or Deglet Noor dates for the best texture and flavor.

- Limit your portion to 2•3 dates per serving, as they are high in natural sugars.

- Pair the dates with a protein•rich food like nuts or nut butter to help slow the absorption of the sugars.

- Dates also make a great addition to smoothies, oatmeal, or baked goods in moderation.

91. Dates (in moderation)

Ingredient:

- 4•6 fresh Medjool or Deglet Noor dates
- Optional toppings:
  - Almond butter or peanut butter
  - Chopped nuts (such as almonds, walnuts, or pecans)
  - Shredded coconut
  - Cinnamon or cocoa powder

Instructions:

1. Wash the dates and pat them dry. Slice them in half lengthwise, or leave them whole if they are small.

2. Arrange the date halves or whole dates on a serving plate or platter.

3. If desired, you can top the dates with any of the following:
   - A small spoonful of almond butter or peanut butter
   - Chopped nuts like almonds, walnuts, or pecans
   - A sprinkle of shredded coconut
   - A light dusting of cinnamon or cocoa powder

That's it! Dates make a naturally sweet and satisfying snack, but they should be consumed in moderation due to their high sugar content.

Dates are a good source of fiber, vitamins, and minerals. The optional toppings can add extra protein, healthy fats, and flavor to balance out the sweetness.

Tips:
- Choose soft, plump Medjool or Deglet Noor dates for the best texture and flavor.
- Limit your portion to 2•3 dates per serving, as they are high in natural sugars.

- Pair the dates with a protein•rich food like nuts or nut butter to help slow the absorption of the sugars.

- Dates also make a great addition to smoothies, oatmeal, or baked goods in moderation.

92. Figs (in moderation)

Ingredient:

- 4-6 fresh figs
- Optional toppings:
  - Honey or agave nectar
  - Crumbled goat or feta cheese
  - Chopped nuts (such as walnuts or pistachios)
  - Balsamic glaze or reduction

Instructions:

1. Wash the figs and pat them dry. Slice the figs in half lengthwise.

2. Arrange the fig halves on a serving plate or platter.

3. If desired, you can top the figs with any of the following:
   - A drizzle of honey or agave nectar
   - Crumbled goat or feta cheese
   - Chopped nuts like walnuts or pistachios
   - A drizzle of balsamic glaze or reduction

That's it! Fresh figs make a naturally sweet and satisfying snack, but they should be consumed in moderation due to their high sugar content.

Figs are a good source of fiber, vitamins, and minerals. The optional toppings can add extra flavor, texture, and nutrients to balance out the sweetness.

Tips:
- Choose ripe, soft figs that are free of blemishes for the best flavor and texture.

- Limit your portion to 2-3 figs per serving, as they are high in natural sugars.

- Pair the figs with a protein-rich food like nuts or cheese to help slow the absorption of the sugars.

- Figs also make a great addition to salads, cheese plates, or baked goods in moderation.

93. Apricot halves

Ingredient:

- 4•6 ripe apricots, halved and pitted
- Optional toppings:
  - Honey or agave nectar
  - Chopped fresh mint or basil
  - Squeeze of lemon or lime juice
  - Crumbled feta or goat cheese

Instructions:

1. Wash the apricots and slice them in half, removing the pits.

2. Arrange the apricot halves on a serving plate or platter.

3. If desired, you can top the apricot halves with any of the following:
   - A drizzle of honey or agave nectar
   - Chopped fresh mint or basil
   - A squeeze of lemon or lime juice
   - Crumbled feta or goat cheese

That's it! Fresh apricot halves make a sweet, juicy, and refreshing snack or dessert.

Apricots have a bright, tangy•sweet flavor that pairs well with the optional toppings. The herbs, citrus, and cheese can add extra layers of flavor and texture.

Tips:
- Choose ripe, soft apricots that are free of blemishes for the best flavor.

- Chill the apricot halves in the refrigerator before serving for maximum refreshment.

- Experiment with different flavor combinations • try drizzling the apricots with a balsamic glaze or sprinkling them with toasted nuts.

- Apricot halves also make a great addition to salads, yogurt parfaits, or as a topping for grilled meats or fish.

94. Sugar•free gelatin

Ingredient:

- 1 (0.25 oz) packet unflavored gelatin
- 1 cup unsweetened fruit juice or water
- 1•2 packets zero•calorie sweetener (such as stevia or erythritol), optional

Instructions:

1. In a small saucepan, sprinkle the gelatin over the fruit juice or water. Let stand for 2•3 minutes to soften the gelatin.

2. Place the saucepan over medium heat and cook, stirring constantly, until the gelatin has completely dissolved, about 2•3 minutes. Do not boil.

3. Remove from heat and stir in the zero•calorie sweetener, if using, until dissolved.

4. Pour the gelatin mixture into a lightly oiled mold or individual ramekins. Refrigerate for at least 4 hours or until set.

5. Once set, run a knife around the edges and invert the gelatin onto a plate or serve in the ramekins.

Tips:
- Use unsweetened fruit juices like apple, grape, or cranberry for more flavor.
- You can also use plain water and add a splash of vanilla extract or lemon juice for flavor.
- Refrigerate any leftover gelatin for up to 5 days.

Enjoy your sugar•free, low•calorie gelatin dessert!

95. Low•fat, sugar•free pudding

Ingredient:

- 2 cups unsweetened almond milk or low•fat milk
- 1/4 cup cornstarch
- 1/4 cup zero•calorie sweetener (such as erythritol or stevia)
- 1/8 teaspoon salt
- 1 teaspoon vanilla extract

Instructions:

1. In a medium saucepan, whisk together the almond milk or low•fat milk, cornstarch, sweetener, and salt until well combined.

2. Place the saucepan over medium heat and cook, stirring constantly, until the mixture thickens and comes to a gentle boil, about 5•7 minutes.

3. Remove the saucepan from the heat and stir in the vanilla extract.

4. Pour the pudding into individual serving dishes or a larger bowl. Cover the surface with plastic wrap to prevent a skin from forming.

5. Refrigerate the pudding for at least 2 hours, or until completely set and chilled.

Tips:
- For a creamier texture, use low•fat milk instead of almond milk.
- You can also add a tablespoon of unsweetened cocoa powder for a chocolate pudding.
- Top with fresh berries, whipped cream, or a sprinkle of cinnamon before serving.
- Store any leftover pudding in the refrigerator for up to 4 days.

Enjoy your low•fat, sugar•free pudding!

96. Chia seed pudding (made with almond milk and stevia)

Ingredient:

- 1 cup unsweetened almond milk
- 3 tablespoons chia seeds
- 1•2 packets of liquid stevia (or to taste)
- 1/2 teaspoon vanilla extract (optional)

Instructions:

1. In a medium bowl, whisk together the almond milk, chia seeds, stevia, and vanilla extract (if using) until well combined.

2. Cover the bowl and refrigerate for at least 4 hours, or overnight, stirring occasionally, until the chia seeds have thickened the mixture into a pudding•like consistency.

3. Serve chilled, either as is or topped with fresh berries, shredded coconut, or a sprinkle of cinnamon.

Tips:
- Start with 1 packet of stevia and add more to taste, depending on your sweetness preference.

- For a thicker pudding, use 4 tablespoons of chia seeds.

- This recipe is perfect for a gastric bypass diet as it is low in calories, high in fiber, and sugar•free.

- The chia seeds provide a good source of protein, healthy fats, and nutrients.

- Chia pudding can be made in advance and stored in the refrigerator for up to 5 days.

Enjoy this delicious and nutritious chia seed pudding that is suitable for a gastric bypass diet!

97. Frozen grapes

Ingredient:

• 1 lb (454g) seedless grapes, washed and dried

Instructions:

1. Carefully remove the grapes from the stem, leaving them in small clusters if desired.

2. Arrange the grapes in a single layer on a baking sheet or plate lined with parchment paper.

3. Place the baking sheet or plate in the freezer and freeze the grapes for at least 2•3 hours, or until completely frozen.

4. Once frozen, transfer the grapes to an airtight container or resealable plastic bag.

5. Store the frozen grapes in the freezer for up to 6 months.

Tips:
• Choose firm, ripe grapes for the best texture when frozen.

• You can freeze different colored grapes (green, red, black) together for a colorful snack.

• Frozen grapes make a great healthy snack or addition to smoothies.

• They can also be used to chill drinks without watering them down as they melt.

• Experiment with different flavors by tossing the grapes in a bit of lemon juice, honey, or cinnamon before freezing.

Enjoy these refreshing and easy•to•make frozen grapes!

98. Low•fat, sugar•free yogurt

Ingredient:

• 4 cups low•fat or nonfat milk
• 2 tablespoons plain Greek yogurt with live active cultures
• 1•2 packets zero•calorie sweetener (such as stevia or erythritol), optional

Instructions:

1. In a medium saucepan, heat the milk over medium heat, stirring occasionally, until it reaches 180°F (82°C). This will help kill any unwanted bacteria.

2. Remove the saucepan from the heat and let the milk cool down to 110•115°F (43•46°C). This temperature is ideal for the yogurt cultures to thrive.

3. In a clean bowl, whisk in the 2 tablespoons of plain Greek yogurt until well combined.

4. Pour the milk•yogurt mixture into a clean container, such as a glass jar or yogurt maker container.

5. Cover the container and incubate the yogurt at 110•115°F (43•46°C) for 6•8 hours, or until the yogurt has thickened to your desired consistency.

6. Once the yogurt has set, stir in the zero•calorie sweetener, if using, to taste.

7. Refrigerate the yogurt for at least 4 hours before serving.

Tips:
• Use low•fat or nonfat milk to keep the yogurt low in fat and calories.
• The longer you incubate the yogurt, the thicker it will become.
• Experiment with different zero•calorie sweeteners to find your preferred taste.
• Top the yogurt with fresh fruit, nuts, or a sprinkle of cinnamon.
• Store the yogurt in the refrigerator for up to 1 week.

Enjoy your homemade, low•fat, sugar•free yogurt!

99. Frozen banana slices

Ingredient:

• 2•3 ripe bananas, peeled and sliced into 1/2•inch thick rounds

Instructions:

1. Line a baking sheet or plate with parchment paper or a silicone baking mat.

2. Arrange the banana slices in a single layer on the prepared surface, making sure they are not touching each other.

3. Place the baking sheet or plate in the freezer and freeze the banana slices for at least 2•3 hours, or until completely frozen.

4. Once frozen, transfer the banana slices to an airtight container or resealable plastic bag.

5. Store the frozen banana slices in the freezer for up to 6 months.

Tips:

• Choose ripe but firm bananas for the best texture when frozen.

• You can dip the banana slices in a bit of lemon juice before freezing to prevent browning.

• Frozen banana slices make a great healthy snack or addition to smoothies.

• They can also be used as a low•calorie, natural sweetener in baked goods or desserts.

• Experiment with different flavors by tossing the banana slices in a bit of cocoa powder, cinnamon, or vanilla extract before freezing.

Enjoy these simple and versatile frozen banana slices!

100. Baked apple with cinnamon

Ingredient:

- 4 medium•sized apples (such as Gala, Honeycrisp, or Fuji)
- 2 tablespoons unsweetened applesauce
- 1 teaspoon ground cinnamon
- 1/4 teaspoon ground nutmeg (optional)
- 2 tablespoons water

Instructions:

1. Preheat your oven to 375°F (190°C).

2. Wash and core the apples, leaving a small well in the center of each one. Be careful not to cut all the way through.

3. In a small bowl, mix together the applesauce, cinnamon, and nutmeg (if using).

4. Place the apples in a baking dish and spoon the cinnamon•applesauce mixture into the center of each apple.

5. Pour the water into the bottom of the baking dish, being careful not to pour it over the apples.

6. Bake the apples for 30•40 minutes, or until they are tender when pierced with a fork.

7. Remove the baked apples from the oven and let them cool for a few minutes before serving.

Tips:
- For a sweeter filling, you can add a teaspoon of honey or maple syrup to the cinnamon•applesauce mixture.

- Serve the baked apples warm, with a dollop of plain Greek yogurt or a sprinkle of chopped nuts on top.

- Leftovers can be stored in the refrigerator for up to 3 days and reheated before serving.

- This recipe is a great healthy dessert or snack option, especially for those following a low•calorie or diabetic•friendly diet.

101. Frozen sugar•free popsicles

Ingredient:

• 2 cups unsweetened fruit juice (such as apple, grape, or cranberry)
• 2 tablespoons zero•calorie sweetener (such as stevia or erythritol)
• 1 tablespoon fresh lemon or lime juice (optional)

Instructions:

1. In a medium bowl, whisk together the fruit juice, zero•calorie sweetener, and lemon or lime juice (if using) until the sweetener is fully dissolved.

2. Carefully pour the sweetened fruit juice mixture into popsicle molds, leaving a small amount of headspace at the top to allow for expansion during freezing.

3. Insert popsicle sticks into the molds, making sure they are centered and secure.

4. Place the popsicle molds in the freezer and freeze for at least 4•6 hours, or until completely solid.

5. Once frozen, gently remove the popsicles from the molds and enjoy immediately.

Tips:
• Use a variety of unsweetened fruit juices to create different flavors of popsicles.

• You can also blend the fruit juice with pureed fruit, such as strawberries or mango, for a creamier texture.

• For a creamy popsicle, substitute 1 cup of the fruit juice with unsweetened almond milk or low•fat milk.

• Experiment with different zero•calorie sweeteners to find your preferred taste.

• Store any leftover popsicles in an airtight container in the freezer for up to 2 months.

Enjoy these refreshing and guilt•free sugar•free popsicles!

102. Low•fat, sugar•free ice cream (in moderation)

Ingredient:

- 2 cups unsweetened almond milk or low•fat milk
- 1/2 cup zero•calorie sweetener (such as erythritol or stevia)
- 2 tablespoons cornstarch
- 1 teaspoon vanilla extract
- Pinch of salt

Instructions:

1. In a medium saucepan, whisk together the almond milk or low•fat milk, sweetener, cornstarch, and salt.

2. Place the saucepan over medium heat and cook, stirring constantly, until the mixture thickens and comes to a gentle boil, about 5•7 minutes.

3. Remove the saucepan from the heat and stir in the vanilla extract.

4. Pour the mixture into a shallow baking dish or metal pan and place it in the freezer.

5. Every 30 minutes, remove the dish from the freezer and stir the mixture with a fork to break up any ice crystals that form. This will help create a smooth, creamy texture.

6. Continue this process for 2•3 hours, or until the ice cream reaches your desired consistency.

7. Once the ice cream is frozen, transfer it to an airtight container and freeze for at least 2 more hours before serving.

Tips:
- For a creamier texture, use low•fat milk instead of almond milk.
- You can also add a tablespoon of vodka or rum to the mixture to help prevent ice crystals from forming.
- Experiment with different zero•calorie sweeteners and flavors, such as chocolate, peanut butter, or mint.
- Scoop the ice cream into individual servings and enjoy in moderation as part of a balanced diet.
- Store the ice cream in the freezer for up to 2 months.

Remember, even though this is a low•fat, sugar•free recipe, ice cream should still be consumed in moderation as part of a healthy lifestyle.

103. Homemade protein bars
(using oats, protein powder, and sugar•free syrup)

Ingredient:

- 2 cups old•fashioned oats
- 1 scoop (about 30g) vanilla or chocolate protein powder
- 1/4 cup sugar•free maple syrup or honey
- 2 tablespoons natural peanut butter or almond butter
- 1/4 cup unsweetened almond milk
- 1/4 teaspoon salt

Optional add•ins:
- 2 tablespoons chopped nuts or seeds
- 2 tablespoons unsweetened shredded coconut
- 1/4 cup dark chocolate chips or cacao nibs

Instructions:

1. Line an 8x8 inch baking pan with parchment paper and set aside.

2. In a large bowl, mix together the oats and protein powder until well combined.

3. In a separate bowl, whisk together the sugar•free syrup, nut butter, almond milk, and salt until smooth.

4. Pour the wet ingredients into the dry ingredients and stir until everything is well incorporated. Fold in any optional add•ins.

5. Press the mixture firmly into the prepared baking pan, using your hands or the back of a spoon to compact it.

6. Refrigerate the bars for at least 2 hours, or until firm.

7. Remove the bars from the pan by lifting the parchment paper. Cut into 8•10 bars. Store the protein bars in an airtight container in the refrigerator for up to 1 week, or in the freezer for up to 3 months.

Tips:
- Use your favorite protein powder flavor, such as chocolate, vanilla, or peanut butter.
- Adjust the amount of sugar•free syrup or honey to your desired sweetness level.
- Customize the bars with your favorite mix•ins, like dried fruit, nuts, or seeds.
- These protein bars are perfect for a quick and healthy snack or post•workout recovery.

104. Sugar•free, low•fat cookies (in moderation)

Ingredient:

• 1 1/2 cups whole wheat flour
• 1/2 cup zero•calorie sweetener (such as erythritol or stevia)
• 1/2 teaspoon baking powder
• 1/4 teaspoon salt
• 1/4 cup unsweetened applesauce
• 2 tablespoons unsweetened almond milk
• 1 teaspoon vanilla extract

Instructions:
1. Preheat your oven to 350°F (175°C). Line a baking sheet with parchment paper.

2. In a medium bowl, whisk together the whole wheat flour, zero•calorie sweetener, baking powder, and salt.

3. In a separate bowl, combine the unsweetened applesauce, almond milk, and vanilla extract.

4. Add the wet ingredients to the dry ingredients and mix until a dough forms. The dough should be slightly sticky but firm.

5. Scoop the dough by the tablespoonful and place the cookies about 2 inches apart on the prepared baking sheet.

6. Bake the cookies for 12•15 minutes, or until they are lightly golden around the edges.

7. Remove the cookies from the oven and let them cool on the baking sheet for 5 minutes before transferring them to a wire rack to cool completely.

Tips:
• For a chewier cookie, use a combination of whole wheat flour and oat flour.
• Add a tablespoon of unsweetened cocoa powder for a chocolate version.
• Stir in a handful of chopped nuts, seeds, or sugar•free chocolate chips for extra flavor and texture.
• Store the cooled cookies in an airtight container at room temperature for up to 5 days.

Remember, even though these cookies are sugar•free and low in fat, they should still be enjoyed in moderation as part of a balanced diet. Portion control is key when it comes to any type of cookie or dessert.

106. Roasted chickpeas

Ingredient:

- 1 (15 oz) can chickpeas (garbanzo beans), drained and rinsed
- 1 tablespoon olive oil
- 1/2 teaspoon ground cumin
- 1/2 teaspoon paprika
- 1/4 teaspoon garlic powder
- 1/4 teaspoon salt
- 1/4 teaspoon black pepper

Instructions:

1. Preheat your oven to 400°F (200°C).

2. Pat the drained and rinsed chickpeas dry with a paper towel or clean kitchen towel.

3. In a medium bowl, toss the chickpeas with the olive oil, cumin, paprika, garlic powder, salt, and black pepper until the chickpeas are evenly coated.

4. Spread the seasoned chickpeas in a single layer on a baking sheet lined with parchment paper.

5. Roast the chickpeas in the preheated oven for 20·25 minutes, stirring halfway, until they are crispy and golden brown.

6. Remove the roasted chickpeas from the oven and let them cool for a few minutes before serving.

Tips:
- For extra crispiness, pat the chickpeas very dry before seasoning and roasting.
- Experiment with different spice blends, such as chili powder, curry powder, or cajun seasoning.
- Roast the chickpeas for a longer time (25·30 minutes) for a crunchier texture.
- Store any leftover roasted chickpeas in an airtight container at room temperature for up to 5 days.
- Enjoy the roasted chickpeas as a healthy snack, salad topping, or addition to soups and stews.

107. Air•popped popcorn (without butter)

Ingredient:

• 1/2 cup unpopped popcorn kernels
• Optional seasonings (such as salt, pepper, garlic powder, etc.)

Instructions:

1. Use an air popper to pop the popcorn kernels. Follow the instructions for your specific air popper model.

2. Once the popcorn is fully popped, transfer it to a large bowl.

3. Season the popcorn with your desired seasonings, if using. Some tasty options include:
• Salt
• Black pepper
• Garlic powder
• Onion powder
• Paprika
• Chili powder
• Nutritional yeast

4. Toss the popcorn gently to evenly distribute the seasonings.

5. Serve the air•popped popcorn immediately while it's hot and fresh.

Tips:
• Avoid using butter or oil, as this will add unnecessary calories and fat.
• Start with 1/2 cup of unpopped kernels, which will yield about 4 cups of popped popcorn.
• Experiment with different seasoning blends to find your favorite flavors.
• Store any leftover popcorn in an airtight container.

Enjoy your healthy, air•popped popcorn snack!

108. Low•fat, whole•grain crackers with low•fat cheese

Ingredient:

• 8•10 whole•grain crackers (look for ones with at least 3g of fiber per serving)
• 1•2 oz low•fat cheese (such as cheddar, mozzarella, or cottage cheese)

Instructions:

1. Select your whole•grain crackers. Look for options that are low in fat and high in fiber, such as:
• Triscuits
• Wasa Crispbread
• Ak•Mak Whole Wheat Crackers
• Finn Crisp Whole Grain Crackers

2. Choose a low•fat cheese variety. Some good options include:
• Low•fat cheddar cheese
• Part•skim mozzarella cheese
• Low•fat cottage cheese

3. Arrange the whole•grain crackers on a plate or platter.

4. Top each cracker with a small slice or spoonful of the low•fat cheese.

5. Serve immediately and enjoy this healthy, protein•packed snack.

Tips:
• Stick to 1•2 oz of cheese per serving to keep the snack low in fat and calories.
• You can also try adding a small amount of fresh herbs, spices, or a drizzle of honey to the cheese for extra flavor.
• This snack provides a good balance of complex carbs, protein, and healthy fats.

109. Rice cakes with low•fat cream cheese and cucumber

Ingredient:

- 2•3 whole grain rice cakes
- 2•3 tbsp low•fat cream cheese
- 1/2 cucumber, sliced

Instructions:

1. Gather your ingredients • whole grain rice cakes, low•fat cream cheese, and fresh cucumber.

2. Spread a thin layer of low•fat cream cheese evenly over the surface of each rice cake.

3. Top the cream cheese with sliced cucumber rounds or strips.

4. Arrange the rice cakes with cucumber on a plate or platter.

That's it! Your healthy snack is ready to enjoy.

Tips:

- Look for rice cakes made with whole grains for more fiber and nutrients.

- Use low•fat or reduced•fat cream cheese to keep the snack lower in calories and fat.

- Slice the cucumber thinly so it lays flat on the rice cakes.

- You can also try adding a sprinkle of black pepper, dill, or other herbs/spices for extra flavor.

- This snack provides a nice balance of complex carbs, protein, and fresh veggies.

110. Whole•grain toast with mashed avocado

Ingredient:

• 2 slices of whole•grain bread or toast
• 1 ripe avocado
• Salt and pepper to taste
• Optional toppings: red pepper flakes, lemon juice, chopped tomatoes, etc.

Instructions:

1. Toast the whole•grain bread until lightly golden brown.

2. In a small bowl, mash the avocado with a fork until it reaches a smooth, spreadable consistency.

3. Spread the mashed avocado evenly over the toasted whole•grain bread slices.

4. Season the avocado toast with a pinch of salt and freshly ground black pepper.

5. If desired, you can also add any additional toppings such as:
• Red pepper flakes for a little spice
• A squeeze of fresh lemon juice for brightness
• Chopped tomatoes or other veggies
• A drizzle of olive oil

6. Serve the whole•grain toast with mashed avocado immediately.

Tips:

• Choose a ripe, soft avocado for the creamiest mashed texture.
• Use 100% whole•grain bread or toast for maximum fiber and nutrients.
• Mash the avocado with a fork or the back of a spoon for a rustic, chunky texture.
• Customize the toppings to your taste preferences.

This simple avocado toast makes for a nutritious and satisfying snack or light meal. Enjoy!

111. Hard•boiled quail eggs

Ingredient:

• 12 quail eggs

Instructions:

1. Gently place the quail eggs in a single layer in a small saucepan. Add enough cold water to the pan to cover the eggs by about 1 inch.

2. Bring the water to a boil over high heat. Once the water reaches a full boil, remove the pan from the heat and cover with a lid.

3. Let the eggs sit in the hot water for 5•6 minutes for a soft•boiled texture, or 7•8 minutes for a hard•boiled texture.

4. Carefully drain the hot water from the pan and cover the eggs with cold water. This will stop the cooking process and make the eggs easier to peel.

5. Let the eggs sit in the cold water for 5•10 minutes.

6. Gently tap each egg against a hard surface to crack the shell, then peel the shells off the eggs.

7. Rinse the peeled hard•boiled quail eggs under cold water to remove any remaining shell fragments.

8. Serve the hard•boiled quail eggs as a snack or use them in other recipes.

Tips:
• Quail eggs are much smaller than chicken eggs, so the cooking time is shorter.
• Be very gentle when peeling the quail eggs, as the shells can be delicate.
• Hard•boiled quail eggs can be stored in the refrigerator for up to 1 week.

Enjoy your healthy, protein•packed quail egg snack!

112. Sliced turkey roll•ups with low•fat cream cheese and spinach

Ingredient:

- 8 oz low•fat cream cheese, softened
- 1 cup fresh spinach leaves, chopped
- 1/4 tsp garlic powder
- 1/4 tsp onion powder
- Salt and pepper to taste
- 8 slices of lean, deli•style turkey breast

Instructions:

1. In a small bowl, mix together the softened low•fat cream cheese, chopped spinach, garlic powder, onion powder, salt, and pepper until well combined.

2. Lay the turkey slices out flat on a clean surface.

3. Spread a thin layer of the cream cheese and spinach mixture evenly over each turkey slice.

4. Carefully roll up each turkey slice, starting from the short end and rolling tightly.

5. Secure the roll•ups with toothpicks, if needed.

6. Slice each roll•up into 2•3 pieces and serve.

Tips:
- Turkey is a lean protein that is easy to digest after gastric bypass surgery.
- The low•fat cream cheese and spinach provide additional nutrients without adding too many calories or fat.
- The simple seasoning adds flavor without the need for high•fat sauces or dressings.
- Serve the turkey roll•ups on their own or with a small side salad for a complete, gastric bypass•friendly meal.
- Be sure to chew the roll•ups thoroughly and eat slowly to prevent discomfort.

Congratulations on exploring the ***"Gastric Bypass Surgery Cookbook: 110+ Nutritious Recipes for Post-Surgery Success."*** This cookbook is dedicated to supporting you on your journey to recovery and wellness after gastric bypass surgery, providing you with over 110 flavorful recipes designed to nourish your body and promote healing.

Navigating life after gastric bypass surgery requires a thoughtful approach to nutrition, focusing on nutrient-dense foods that support your health and well-being. Each recipe in this cookbook has been carefully crafted to prioritize protein, vitamins, and minerals essential for your recovery journey. From satisfying breakfasts to comforting dinners and everything in between, these recipes are tailored to help you maintain a balanced diet while adjusting to your new lifestyle.

We understand that the path to recovery can have its challenges, and our hope is that this cookbook has empowered you with practical meal ideas and nutritional guidance. By embracing a diet rich in lean proteins, vegetables, and wholesome ingredients, you are not only supporting your physical health but also setting the stage for long-term success and vitality.

As you continue to explore the recipes in this cookbook, we encourage you to listen to your body, celebrate your progress, and savor the journey of healing and renewal. Remember, each meal is an opportunity to nourish yourself and support your recovery goals.

*We sincerely hope that the **"Gastric Bypass Surgery Cookbook"** becomes a trusted companion on your path to post-surgery success. May these recipes inspire you, bring joy to your table, and contribute to your overall well-being as you embrace a healthier, more fulfilling life.*

Thank you for choosing this cookbook to support your journey. Here's to your health, happiness, and a future filled with delicious, nutritious meals that support your ongoing recovery and well-being.

Wishing you all the best on your continued journey of health and healing.

Bon appétit!